Recent Results in Cancer Research 102

Recent Results in Cancer Research

Volume 95: Spheroids in Cancer Research
Edited by H. Acker, J. Carlsson, R. Durand, R. M. Sutherland
1984. 83 figures, 12 tables. IX, 183. ISBN 3-540-13691-6

Volume 96: Adjuvant Chemotherapy of Breast Cancer
Edited by H.-J. Senn
1984. 98 figures, 91 tables. X, 243. ISBN 3-540-13738-6

Volume 97: Small Cell Lung Cancer
Edited by S. Seeber
1985. 44 figures, 47 tables. VII, 166. ISBN 3-540-13798-X

Volume 98: Perioperative Chemotherapy
Edited by U. Metzger, F. Largiadèr, H.-J. Senn
1985. 48 figures, 45 tables. XII, 157. ISBN 3-540-15124-9

Volume 99: Peptide Hormones in Lung Cancer
Edited by K. Havemann, G. Sorenson, C. Gropp
1985. 100 figures, 63 tables. XII, 248. ISBN 3-540-15504-X

Volume 100:
Therapeutic Strategies in Primary and Metastatic Liver Cancer
Edited by Ch. Herfarth, P. Schlag, P. Hohenberger
1986. 163 figures, 104 tables. ISBN 3-540-16011-6

Volume 101:
Locoregional High-Frequency Hyperthermia and Temperature Measurements
Edited by G. Bruggmoser, W. Hinkelbein, R. Engelhardt, M. Wannenmacher
1986. 96 figures, 8 tables. IX, 143. ISBN 3-540-15501-5

Epidemiology of Malignant Melanoma

Edited by R. P. Gallagher

With 15 Figures and 70 Tables

Springer-Verlag
Berlin Heidelberg New York Tokyo

Richard P. Gallagher, M. A.

Cancer Control Agency of British Columbia
600 West 10th Avenue
Vancouver, B. C. V5Z 4E6, Canada

ISBN-13:978-3-642-82643-6 e-ISBN-13:978-3-642-82641-2
DOI: 10.1007/978-3-642-82641-2

Library of Congress Cataloging-in-Publication Data. Main entry under title: Epidemiology of malignant melanoma. (Recent results in cancer research; v. 102) Based on a conference held in Vancouver in 1984, sponsored by the Cancer Control Agency of British Columbia. Includes bibliographies and index. 1. Melanoma-Congresses. 2. Carcinogenesis-Congresses. 3. Epidemiology-Congresses. 4. Environmentally induced diseases-Congresses. I. Gallagher, R. P. (Richard P.), 1944- . II. Cancer Control Agency of British Columbia. III. Series. [DNLM: 1. Melanoma-etiology-congresses. 2. Melanoma-occurrence-congresses. W1 RE106P v. 102/QZ 202 E639 1984] RC261.R35 vol. 102 616.99'4 [616.99'4071] 85-27796[RC280.S5]

2125/3140-543210

Preface

Interest in the etiology of malignant melanoma has increased enormously in the last 10 years, after it was realized that the incidence of the cutaneous form of the disease was rising.

Treatment of the disease has not improved dramatically, and our best hope for curtailing the rise in mortality and morbidity from the disease appears to be primarily through early detection and, perhaps in the future, through prevention. It is thus very important for the medical community to be able to recognize individuals and groups at high risk of the disease because of either familial and constitutional factors and lifestyle or exposure to environmental risk factors.

This book, arising from a meeting held in Vancouver in 1984, provides a summary of the latest findings among Caucasian populations along with perspectives on the most important environmental risk factors identified to date. Comparison of results from the four major analytic studies presented here also demonstrates that a number of factors implicated in other common cancers are probably not related to the incidence of melanoma. These include smoking, alcohol consumption, and for the most part, diet.

The Vancouver conference was sponsored by the Cancer Control Agency of British Columbia, and was financially supported by Health and Welfare Canada (6610-1429-50), the Northern California Cancer Program (NCCP), Miles Laboratories (Canada), Bristol Myers Laboratories (Canada), and Plough Canada Inc.

I owe a special debt of gratitude to Mrs. Shirley Morton and in particular to Mrs. Jean van den Broek, who managed most of the details of the meeting and typed the manuscripts.

Vancouver, December 1985 Richard P. Gallagher

Contents

*List of Contributors**

Armstrong, B.K. *18*[1]
Austin, D.F. *98*
Bain, C. *76*
Bale, S.J. *144*
Blackwell, J.B. *18*
Cumming, F.J. *18*
Dubin, N. *56*
Duray, P.H. *154*
Elwood, J.M. *38, 127, 137*
English, D.R. *18*
Ernstoff, M. *154*
Gallagher, R.P. *38*
Green, A. *76*
Greene, M.H. *144*
Hartge, P. *159*
Hill, G.B. *38*
Heenan, P.J. *18*
Holland, S. *18*
Holly, E.A. *108, 118*
Holman, C.D.J. *18*
Kelsall, G.R.H. *18*
Kirkwood, J.M. *154*
Klaus, S.N. *154*
Lerner, A.B. *154*
Matz, L.R. *18*
Maxwell, K.J. *137*
McLennan, R. *76*
Møller Jensen, O. *8*
Moseson, M. *56*
Østerlind, A. *8*
Pasternack, B.S. *56*
Reynolds, P. *98*
Rouse, I.L. *18*
Roush, G.C. *154*
Shields, J.A. *159*
Singh, A. *18*
Siskind, V. *76*
Somma, S.J. *154*
Stenn, K.S. *154*
Ten Seldam, R.E.J. *18*
Titus, L.J. *154*
Tucker, M.A. *159*
Watt, J.D. *18*
Worth, A.J. *1*
Xu, Z. *18*

---

* The address of the principal author is given on the first page of each contribution

[1] Page on which contribution begins

Pathology of Melanoma

Growth Patterns in Melanoma and Its Precursor Lesions

A. J. Worth

Head of Clinical Laboratories, Cancer Control Agency of British Columbia, 600 West 10th Avenue, Vancouver, B.C. V5Z 4E6, Canada

In this presentation on the pathology of malignant melanoma I would like to consider briefly some of growth patterns which are seen in melanomata and in associated melanocytic precursor lesions. I shall attempt to relate the growth patterns to the biology of the disease and to the clinical presentation.

Malignant melanoma appears to be increasing in incidence, the rate of increase in Canada exceeding that for every other tumor except lung cancer, while in southern Arizona the incidence increased by 340% between 1969 and 1978 (Fitzpatrick et al. 1985). Fortunately, many melanomata are detected at an earlier stage, but late, deeply invasive lesions are still frequently seen. Although the clinical features of dysplastic nevi and other precursor lesions are becoming more sharply defined and the role of ultraviolet radiation is under intense study, we are still not capable of determining who is actually at risk for developing a melanoma with sufficient accuracy to develop adequate screening programs. At present the detection of dysplastic nevi and early malignant transformation depends upon clinical recognition of the lesion.

The cell of concern is, of course, the melanocyte. It is thought that the melanocytic precursor cells migrate from the neural crest to the skin and other parts of the body very early in life, melanocytes being found in the epidermis by the third month of fetal development. In the adult skin the melanocyte is seen as a small dendritic cell with clear cytoplasm, which is located singly in the basal portions of the epidermis adjacent to the epithelial basement membrane. The melanocyte is characterized by the presence of tyrosinase and melanosomes, which differentiate it from the dendritic Langerhans' cells and intermediate cells which may also be found within the epidermis. The melanosome, which is the specific granule of the melanocyte, is found singly within the functional melanocyte, but when transferred through the dendritic cytoplasm of the melanocyte to the adjacent epithelial cells, the granules are aggregated into membrane-bound organelles, which may be visible in tissue sections as melanin granules. In melanomas and in other melanocytic dysplasias the melanosomes may assume an abnormal structure, or they may be absent in amelanotic clones.

In future, with the advent of monoclonal antibodies, we may no longer have to depend upon morphological characteristics to identify melanocytes and to evaluate melanocytic disorders. Antimelanoma antibodies are already on the market, and they offer exciting prospects for the future. An antibody which has already proved to be most useful in distinguishing melanocytes from other connective tissue cells and from epithelial cells is S100 protein.

Recent Results in Cancer Research. Vol 102

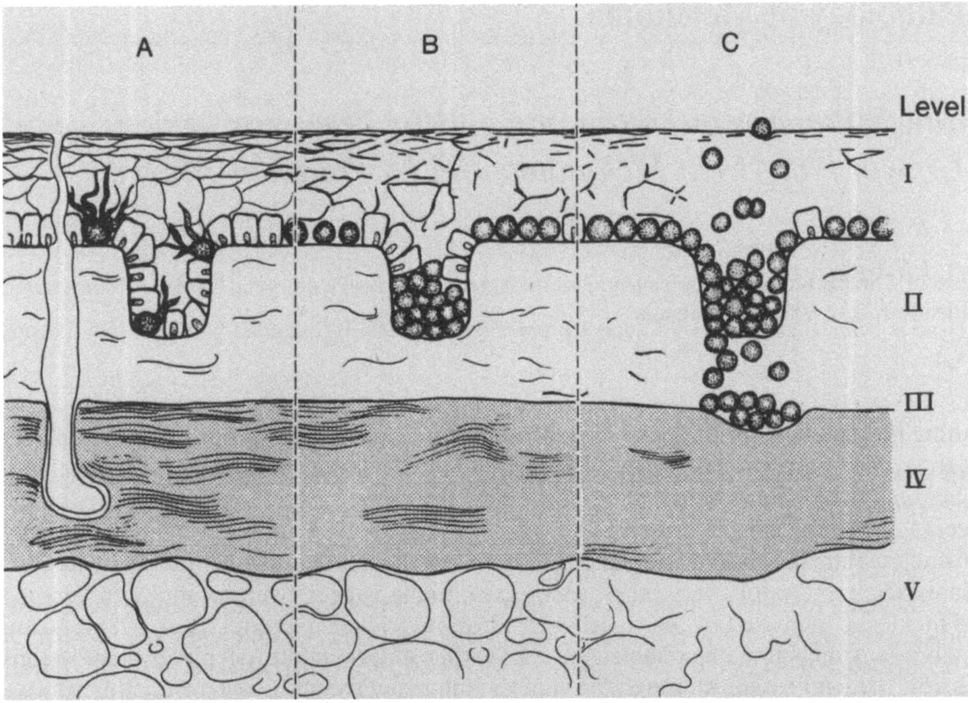

Fig. 1 A–C. Patterns of melanocytic proliferation. **A** Normal melanocytes growing as dendritic cells, distributed along the basement membrane and interdigitating between the basal epithelial cells. **B** A numeric abnormality is seen, the melanocytes being increased in number. There also is a positional abnormality, as the melanocytes are clustering and becoming confluent in one of the rete pegs. **C** Numeric and positional abnormalities are present, with the melanocytes (in addition to showing confluent growth along the basement membrane) demonstrating upward invasion through the epidermis to the keratin layer. Melanocytes have broken through the basement membrane and are accumulating at and pressing against the papillary reticular dermal border. This growth pattern represents an invasive level III melanoma.
Levels: *I*, cells confined to the epithelium above the basement membrane; *II*, malignant cells invading the papillary dermis; *III*, malignant cells reach and accumulate at the papillary-reticular dermal border; *IV*, invasion of the reticular dermis; *V*, invasion of the subcutaneous tissues

When looking at a section of normal skin one may have considerable difficulty in identifying normal melanocytes, for as mentioned previously, they are small cells tucked along the basal layers of the epithelium. Although they are scattered throughout the entire skin surface they are most numerous along the basal portions of the rete pegs of the epidermis. In many melanocytic disorders the number, distribution, and localization of melanocytic cells within the epidermis may be of considerable help in arriving at the correct diagnosis and can be of assistance in the understanding of the malignant potential of the lesion.

Melanocytic lesions, therefore, may be viewed in terms of the numerical, positional, and morphological and/or cytological abnormalities which may be present. Generally speaking, the presence of a numerical increase in the number of cells in the absence of a positional or cytological aberration is the least significant perturbation, the positional and cytological abnormalities generally being associated with dysplasias and malignancy (Fig. 1). In the most innocuous lesions, such as freckles and lentigines, the prominence of the cells in the rete ridges is lost, so that the proliferating melanocytes come to form a discontinuous layer with the cells randomly distributed along the basement membrane. This pattern is associated also with lentigo maligna, but in this lesion the melanocytes come to form a confluent layer along the basement membrane. In lentiginous types of dysplasia and in lentigo maligna, the numerical and positional abnormalities of melanocytic growth are also accompanied by individual cellular atypia with nuclear enlargement and nuclear cytoplasmic abnormalities.

In other lesions the melanocytes may not only increase in number and become confluent, but may tend to migrate from the basal portions of the epithelium up through the epidermis to the surface. In other words, the cells are demonstrating local invasive capabilities deviating from their normal position. This is the pattern seen in dysplastic nevi and in superficial spreading malignant melanoma.

In comparing these prior two growth patterns, it seems reasonable to assume that the cells that retain their normal position are probably under better biological control than those that are migrating upwards or infiltrating deeply into adjacent tissues. One might make a shrewd guess that a comparison between the biology of the two types of lesions would show that the "infiltrative" pattern was the more aggressive of the two. The cells, of course, may not multiply singly, but rather aggregate into small nests or groups, which may remain at the basement, transgress the epidermis, or form small clusters which eventually drop off the basement membrane and invade the underlying connective tissue (Fig. 1).

It is by an analysis of the deviations from the normal growth pattern that the pathologist is able to identify and classify the various melanocytic lesions.

Benign Nevi

In the actively growing benign nevus, nests of cells are usually found in the junctional position adjacent to the basement membrane. When these cells, in the natural evolution of the lesion, drop off the basement membrane and extend into the underlying dermis, they usually cease to divide and become small inactive mature cells which only rarely undergo malignant transformation. In contrast to the benign maturing compound or intradermal nevus, some of the larger persistent congenital nevi tend to be composed of single cells, which may extend deep into the dermis and subcutaneous tissue, particularly in association with adnexal structures. It is thought that congenital nevi, particularly those in excess of 2 cm in diameter, carry with them a higher risk for the development of malignancy later in life.

Some melanocytic nevi, such as Spitz nevi, spindle cell nevi, and active melanocytic nevi in the vulval area in young women, may give rise to difficulties in interpretation, because the nevus cells demonstrate both positional and cytological abnormalities with enlarged nuclei and prominent nucleoli. In addition, they may fail to demonstrate maturation, with the intradermal nevus cells remaining mitotically active. In such lesions, the overall symmetry of the proliferative process and the lack of a single cell infiltrative pattern within the epidermis may be clues to the benign characteristics of the lesion. To assess these lesions adequately it is important that the clinical presentation and the overall growth pattern of the lesion be taken into consideration. It can easily by appreciated that a small punch biopsy may be misleading in such a context. Complete excision biopsy is preferable, as this permits evaluation of the symmetry of the growth of the entire tumor.

Dysplastic Nevi

Premalignant melanocytic dysplasia have only become clearly defined in the last few years (Ackerman and Mihara 1985). The recognition of these lesions and their distinction from active junctional compound nevi and Spitz nevi has led to a better understanding of the biology of malignant melanomata and to the identification of high-risk individual patients as well as high-risk families. Dysplastic nevi may demonstrate an unstable continued growth, with a significant number of cases evolving into in situ and invasive malignant melanomata. The dysplastic nevus clinically has a characteristic appearance, with irregular margins and uneven pigmentation, which is characterized pathologically by an abnormal and frequently diffuse proliferation of melanocytic cells along the basal layer. They may present a varied appearance, being composed of small inconspicuous cells as well as large atypical spindle and epithelioid melanocytes. Even in early stages of development, when they may display only mild cytological atypia, the nevi are frequently underlain by an expanded and abnormal papillary dermis within which there is focal proliferation of fibroblasts, proliferation of small capillary channels, and a mild to marked inflammatory host response chiefly of lymphocytes. These changes in the dermis suggest that during the period of evolution the melanocytic cells are undergoing subtle molecular changes, possibly evolving new and abnormal membrane antigens which are responsible for eliciting the host response. The pathological diagnosis of a dysplastic nevus is based therefore upon the presence of both numerical and positional abnormalities of melanocytic proliferation, while the degree of dysplasia correlates with the extent of the nuclear cytoplasmic cellular atypia.

In a fashion analogous to dysplasias involving other organs, such as the cervix, dysplastic nevi may progress slowly over many years, or rapidly into melanoma in situ and invasive disease. Some may remain static, failing to progress through a patient's life span. With the onset of transepidermal invasion and increasing cellular atypia, the lesion is recognized as a melanoma in situ. Dysplastic nevi occurring in sporadic fashion are thought to undergo malignant transformation in about 10% of patients; whereas for those patients who have a family history, in particular with two or more relatives with dysplastic nevi, it is thought that during their life span they are almost certain to develop malignant melanoma (Elder et al. 1981; National Institutes of Health 1984).

Malignant Melanoma

As alluded to previously, the classification of malignant melanoma is based on the pattern of intraepidermal growth. In lentigo maligna melanoma, the characteristic pattern is that of a confluent proliferation of abnormal melanocytes along the basal layer, whereas superficial spreading malignant melanomas are characterized by transepidermal migration of viable malignant cells upwards into the keratin layer, either singly of in irregularly distributed nests of large, clear, nucleolated and mitotic, active malignant cells. These melanomata appear to remain confined to the epidermis for long periods of time, demonstrating first a lateral spreading growth pattern prior to acquiring the capability to invade and survive within the underlying dermis which is referred to as the vertical growth phase. In situ malignant melanomata are frequently underlain by an intense inflammatory host response and may demonstrate lack of definition of the basement membrane. Examination by electron microscopy of the in situ malignancies frequently demonstrates that there is migration by individual cells through the basement membrane over a long period of time.

These cells, although they are capable of invading the dermis, have not acquired the capacity to survive within the stroma. They initially die out, being destroyed by the host response. Eventually, however, perhaps due to a process of clonal selection, a clone of cells may evolve which is capable of surviving within the host tissues. This process of clonal selection is not well understood. It may evolve rapidly, or only after many years of in situ proliferation; or it may never evolve at all. At the present time we are unable to predict the subsequent behavior of an individual dysplastic lesion. During the process of clonal selection, it appears that antigenic changes take place in the cell membranes of the evolving melanoma cells, the vertical growth phase being frequently associated with less well differentiated cells, increased mitotic activity, minimal or absent host response, and decreased melanin pigmentation.

In an attempt to quantitate the risk of subsequent development of metastatic disease, numerous parameters of invasive melanoma have been examined. The clinical stage is of the greatest predictive value, followed by micrometer measurement of the depth of invasion of the melanoma, and by levelling (Balch et al. 1981). In assessment of the level of invasion, the location of the deepest malignant melanocytic cell within the dermis is related to the normal dermal structure. Normal skin contains a very thin papillary dermis characterized by loose fine bundles of collagen and a relatively small number of lymphatics. Underlying the papillary dermis is the reticular dermis, which is characterized by coarse collagen bundles, adnexal structures and increased numbers of larger lymphatic vessels and nerves. A level I melanoma refers to an in situ malignant melanoma in which all the cells are found confined to the epidermis above the basement membrane (Fig. 1). A level II lesion refers to those melanomata in which the cells are found within the papillary dermis. Level III indicates a lesion in which the cells have reached the papillary reticular dermal border and are accumulating at and pressing against the border, but not yet significantly infiltrating the underlying reticular dermis. Level IV is associated with reticular dermal invasion and level V, with involvement of subcutaneous tissue. Thickness of the skin varies from one area of the body to another, so that the level may not reflect the actual depth of invasion. Micrometer measurement of the depth of invasion gives a more accurate measurement when coupled with a measurement of the transverse diameter of the lesion, and the two values give a better assessment of the total volume of malignant cells which are present, and are generally felt to constitute an individual parameter that correlates better with prognosis than the level of invasion.

Recently, it has been recognized that the degree of cellular variability of the invasive component, the mitotic rate and the growth pattern – whether it be spindle, epithelioid or clustered – are significant prognostic indicators (Day et al. 1982). This type of classification does seem to make sense, for some melanomata appear highly aggressive, being markedly pleomorphic and mitotic, in contrast to others that may be composed of cells that are extremely bland and uniform with little mitotic activity, although both lesions may be of equal depth and size. Those lesions which demonstrate little individual cellular abnormality and which have a favorable prognosis with low metastatic potential are classified as borderline lesions.

Nodular Melanoma

There are some melanomata which, from their inception, appear to become rapidly invasive without a prolonged lateral spreading in situ growth phase. When examining these lesions one may be unable to detect a marginal in situ component. Such lesions are classified as nodular malignant melanomata. The frequency with which such lesions are diagnosed will vary with the care with which the lesion is sectioned in an attempt to demonstrate a marginal in situ component.

Lentigo Maligna Melanoma

Lentigo maligna melanoma is the name applied to the lesions usually found in elderly patients on the face or hand. There is continuous proliferation of abnormal melanocytic cells along the basal layer. In its original stages this change may be subtle, with only occasional abnormal mitoses and minimal transepidermal migration. As the disease progresses, the changes may come to more closely resemble those seen in superficial spreading malignant melanoma. The invasive nodules which develop within these lesions may be quite indolent.

Acral Lentiginous Melanoma

The acral lentiginous melanomata of the soles of the feet and the palms of the hand as well as the mucosal melanomas may display a similar life cycle. In the in situ phase these lesions are characterized by the proliferation of small, relatively inconspicuous pale melanocytic cells with a confluent growth pattern and partial transepidermal migration. While fairly characteristic, this pattern may at times be indistinguishable from a superficial spreading or lentigo maligna melanoma. The mucosal melanomas are of particular interest, as clearly they cannot be directly attributable to sun exposure. A different etiology has to be invoked.

Regression

Regression is a phenomenon which is seen fairly frequently in malignant melanomata, but seldom in other malignancies. In superficial spreading melanoma, in particular, one may see stromal changes comprising an expanded, fibrosed, vascularized, and inflamed papillary or papillary and superficial reticular dermis in which there may be still a few residual viable or dying melanoma cells. Varying degrees of regression may be seen in different areas of an individual lesion. In some instances, the primary may regress entirely even in the presence of actively growing metastatic disease. If we knew what triggered this mechanism, useful information for the management of both primary and metastatic disease might be available.

Clinical Recognition of Melanocytic Lesions

While the previously described growth patterns form the basis for pathological classification of melanoma, the understanding of the biology of the disease also facilitates the clinical interpretation of melanocytic lesions. A small symmetrical pigmented lesion in which the pigment is uniform and which is covered by uniform and intact surface epithelium has all the clinical hallmarks of a benign lesion. On the other hand, the lesion with irregular margins, with irregular pigmentation, demonstrating a lateral spreading growth pattern, is consistent with a dysplastic or malignant melanocytic proliferation in which numerical, positional, and clonal differences might be anticipated within the proliferating cells. The presence of scaling, crusting, or oozing would be associated with transepidermal migration of the malignant cells, and itching with an inflammatory infiltrate. Developing pallor and flattening of the lesion might indicate regression, while a pale pink or white nodule developing within the pigmented lesion would indicate the evolution of an amelanotic clone. A nodular, sharply demarked lesion without a lateral spreading area of pigmentation might typify a nodular melanoma. Palpability or elevation usually correlates with the presence of a vertical growth phase and dermal invasion.

From this brief review of the pathology of melanocytic lesions it is apparent that the clinical presentation and prognosis reflects their biological growth pattern.

References

Ackerman AB, Mihara I (1985) Dysplasia, dysplastic melanocytes, dysplastic nevi, the dysplastic nevus syndrome, and the relation between dysplastic nevi and malignant melanomas. Hum Pathol 16: 87–91

Balch CM, Soong SJ, Murad TM, Ingalls AL, Maddox WA (1981) A multifactorial analysis of melanoma: III. Prognostic factors in melanoma patients with lymph node metastases (stage II). Ann Surg 193: 377–388

Day CL, Harrist TJ, Lew RA, Mihm MC Jr (1982) Classification of malignant melanoma according to the histologic morphology of melanoma nodules. J Dermatol Surg Oncol 8: 874–875, 900

Elder DE, Greene MH, Bondi EF, Clark WH Jr (1981) Acquired melanocytic nevi and melanoma. In: Ackerman AB (ed) Pathology of malignant melanoma. Masson, New York, pp 185–216

Fitzpatrick TB, Rhodes AR, Sober AJ (1985) Prevention of melanoma by recognition of its precursors. (Letter) N Engl J Med 312: 1388

National Institutes of Health (1984) Precursors to malignant melanoma. National Institutes of Health Consensus Development Conference Statement, October 24–26, 1983. J Am Acad Dermatol 10: 683–688

Descriptive and Analytic Studies of Cutaneous Melanoma

Trends in Incidence of Malignant Melanoma of the Skin in Denmark 1943–1982

A. Østerlind and O. Møller Jensen

Danish Cancer Registry, Institute of Cancer Epidemiology Under the Danish Cancer Society, Landskronagade 66, 2100 Copenhagen Ø, Denmark

Introduction

Malignant melanoma of the skin is largely confined to Caucasians, and it is especially frequent in countries with fair-skinned populations (Crombie 1979b; Waterhouse et al. 1982). Ultraviolet light from the sun seems to play a dominant role as a risk factor; white skin lacks the protection against ultraviolet light that pigmented people acquire from melanin in the basal layer of the epidermis (Crombie 1979a). The differences observed between more and less developed white societies and between people living in Scandinavia and in the Mediterranean countries may arise because even minor differences in the natural pigmentation of the skin play a major role in the risk of cutaneous melanoma. To what extent the considerable increases in the incidence of skin melanomas observed in some white populations (Jensen and Bolander 1980; Little et al. 1980; Magnus 1977) are related to changes in habits and general way of life and how much protection pigmentation provides against the influence of a more hazardous, opulent life-style must still be investigated. Clarification and recognition of relations between life-style and risk of malignant melanoma may ultimately result in public counselling with the aim of reversing the steadily increasing health problems caused by this malignancy.

Efforts to clarify the epidemiology of melanoma, especially in high-risk areas, have therefore been intensified within the last decade. Analysis of cancer registry data provides essential information on trends and on quantitative aspects of risk in various groups of the population. Descriptive studies are now being supplemented with analytical investigations in which individuals are characterized with regard to both presence of malignant melanoma and putative risk factors. This paper presents an analysis of data on cutaneous melanoma cases in Denmark, reported to the Danish Cancer Registry from 1943 to 1982.

Materials and Methods

Since 1943 the national Danish Cancer Registry has registered all cases of cancer occurring in the Danish population. The registration system is based on notifications from all clinical and pathology departments of Danish hospitals and practicing physicians (mainly dermatologists) and is supplemented with information from death certificates. Reporting is voluntary, and recent evaluations indicate that cancer registration may for all practical purposes be regarded as complete and valid (Østerlind and Jensen 1985). All new cases of

Recent Results in Cancer Research. Vol 102

cancer since 1943 have been categorized according to an extended version of the Seventh Revision of the International Classification of Diseases, and the coding is carried out by trained nosologists.

The present investigation includes all incident cases of malignant melanoma of the skin. Metastatic malignant melanomas from unknown primary tumors are not included (275 cases); the tabulation of the material affects primarily the latter half of the 40-year period. The diagnosis was histologically verified in 98% of the cases in the latest period from 1973 to 1980, whereas only 83% of the cases were verified inthe period 1943-1952 (Clemmesen 1965; Danish Cancer Registry 1982, 1983). The incidence rates are presented for the period 1943-1982, whereas the mortality rates are only available from 1955 to 1982. All incidence and mortality rates are average annual rates per 100000 persons, with the average annual Danish population of the period as denominator. Age is standardized by the direct method to the world standard population (Waterhouse et al. 1976).

Information on anatomic site is available for nearly all cases, and the definition of site is unchanged from 1943 to 1982. The tumors have been grouped by anatomic site as follows: head and face (including scalp), neck and trunk, upper limb, lower limb, and other and unspecified [including malignant melanomas (MM) of multiple sites, MM with unspecified anatomic location, and MM of anus].

Results

This investigation comprises a total of 8814 cases, 3509 male and 5305 female patients, with malignant melanoma of the skin in Denmark, diagnosed between 1943 and 1982. During this period the average annual number of incident cases has increased from around 50 cases in 1943 to 470 cases in 1982 (Fig. 1). The age-standardized incidence rates have shown a five- to sixfold increase for both sexes (Fig. 2). The increase has been most pronounced since 1955, and at present there is no indication of levelling off. Females clearly exceed males in incidence rate during the entire period. The female-to-male ratio

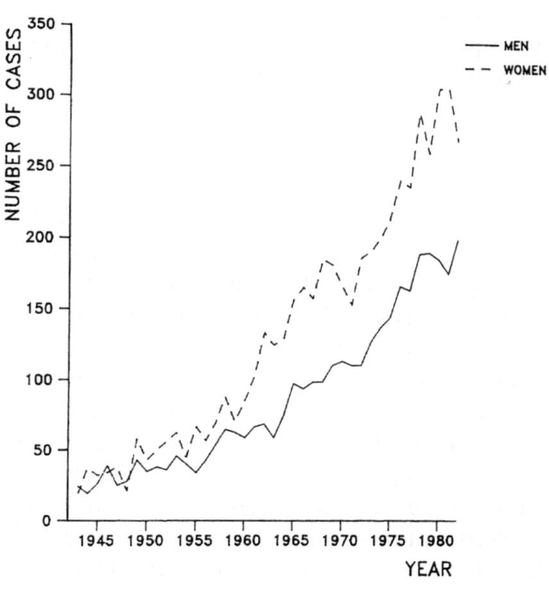

Fig. 1. Annual number of new cases of malignant melanoma of the skin in Denmark 1943-1982

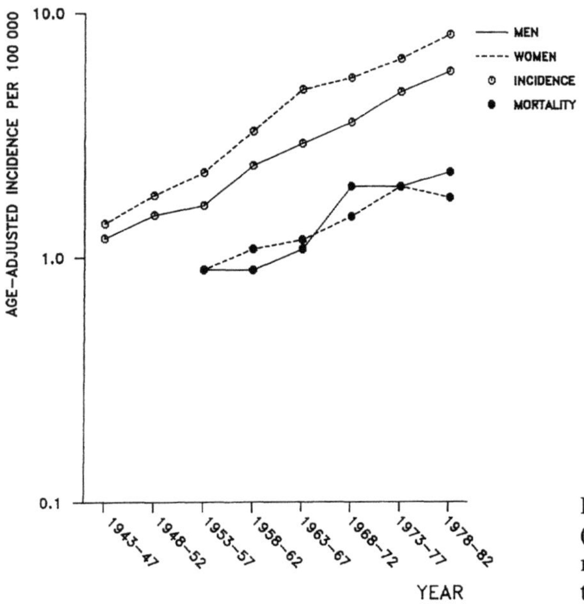

Fig. 2. Average annual age-standardized (world standard) incidence rates and mortality rates of malignant melanoma of the skin in Denmark 1943-1982

Table 1. Average annual age-standardized incidence per 100000 (world standard) and female-to-male ratio of malignant melanoma of the skin in Denmark 1943-1982

Time period	Male	Female	Ratio
1943-1947	1.20	1.38	1.15
1948-1952	1.50	1.81	1.21
1953-1957	1.65	2.26	1.37
1958-1962	2.42	3.34	1.38
1963-1967	2.99	4.99	1.67
1968-1972	3.66	5.59	1.53
1973-1977	4.91	6.71	1.37
1978-1982	5.99	8.48	1.42

of 1.15 in 1943-1947 rose to a maximum of 1.67 in 1963-1967, whereas the last decade seems to reflect stabilization at al level of 1.40 (Table 1).

The age-standardized mortality rate for the period 1955-1982 is also included in Fig. 2. The mortality rate doubled during this period, but the rate of increase did not start to accelerate in either men or women until 1965 - a decade after the acceleration of the incidence rates. The tendency of a levelling among women since 1975 is also seen 10 years after the break in the incidence curve. In recent years the mortality rate has been highest in male patients in spite of the observed higher female incidence rate throughout the period.

The change over time in the incidence rates has differed between various anatomic sites and between the sexes (Figs. 3 and 4). The increase among males has been most marked for tumors of the trunk, with a ten-fold increase during the period 1943-1982, followed by lower limb and upper limb, in both of which the incidence has increased around

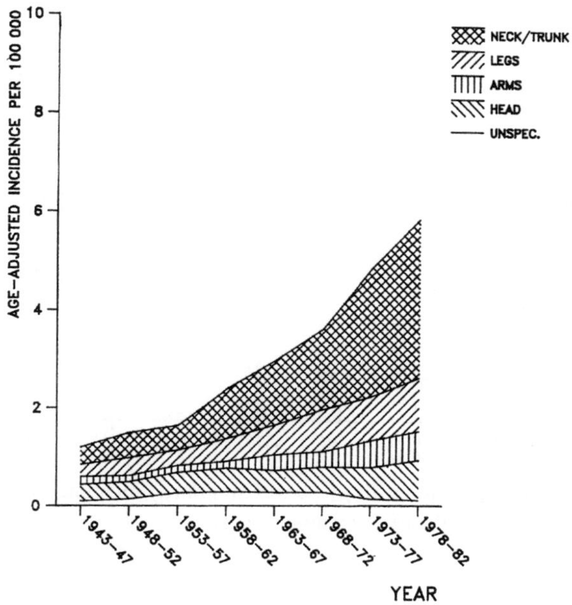

Fig. 3. Age-standardized (world standard) male incidence rates of malignant melanoma of the skin in Denmark 1943-1982, by anatomic site

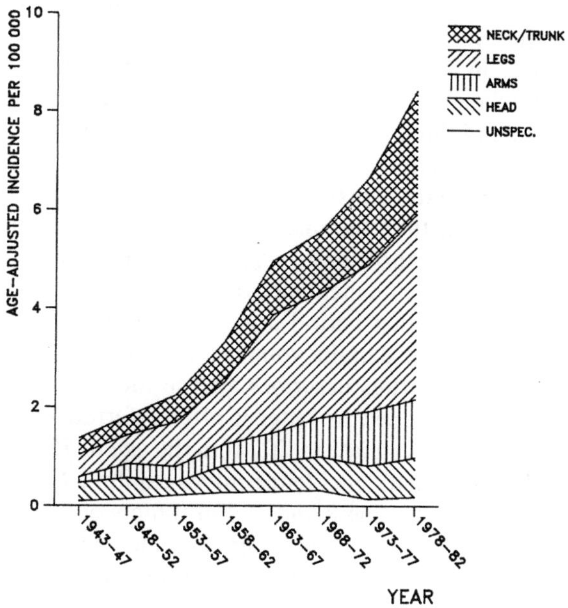

Fig. 4. Age-standardized (world standard) female incidence rates of malignant melanoma of the skin in Denmark 1943-1982, by anatomic site

four times (Fig. 3). Among women the most pronounced increase is seen for tumors of the lower limb, with an eight-fold increase, followed by almost similar proportional increases for melanomas located on the trunk and the upper limb (Fig. 4). Only relatively minor changes have been observed in the incidence of melanoma of the head, which doubled. In male patients more than 60% of the increase in the total incidence was attributable to tumors of the trunk followed by tumors on the lower limb (18%). In female patients the in-

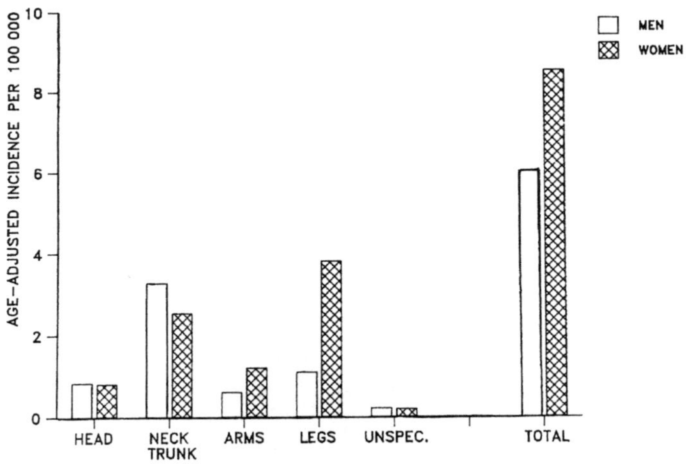

Fig. 5. Age-standardized (world standard) incidence rates of malignant melanoma of the skin in Denmark 1978-1982, by anatomic site

crease in incidence rate for melanoma of the lower limb constituted 47% of the total increase, followed by tumors on the trunk (31%). In the latest period the most marked increase is seen for malignant melanomas of the trunk and neck in female patients.

The overall age-standardized rates by site for the most recent 5-year period 1978-1982 is given in Fig. 5. Among males the most common location is the trunk, which accounts for 55% of melanomas, followed by the lower limb with 18%. In women the lower limbs (47%) and the trunk (30%) are the sites most often affected. Male preponderance is seen for the incidence of melanoma of the trunk, whereas an excess is seen for lower limb in female patients. The female incidence rate of melanoma of lower limb is more than three times higher than the male rate. An excess incidence among female patients is also observed for the upper limb, whereas for the head there is no difference between the sexes.

The age-specific incidence rates for four successive 10-year periods are shown in Figs. 6 and 7. In the first period a gradual increase with age is observed. Due to a more pronounced increase in the younger and middle age groups the curve has changed. The current incidence thus describes a steep increase from 20 to 50 years of age, followed by a more gentle slope (the latter is often referred to as a plateau). Among men a further increase is observed late in life from the age of 75 years onward.

The age-specific incidence curves exhibit a different course for tumors at different anatomic locations (Figs 8 and 9). For tumors of the head in both sexes the incidence rate increases exponentially with age. For melanoma of the head the incidence rate changed little in successive time periods, although an increased incidence rate is observed for males in the most recent time period. This increase seemed to take place 10 years earlier in women. The age-specific incidence of melanoma of the trunk in both sexes and of melanoma of the lower limb in girls and women showed a steep increase starting in adolescence and continuing to middle age, after which the incidence showed a levelling off. The male excess in the risk of melanoma of the trunk is apparent in all time periods and all age groups except for the most recent time period, where female subjects under 35 years have been more at risk than men. The female excess for tumors on the lower limb is apparent in all time periods and in all age groups. In female patients the increase in risk for all sites together was highest in the 20- to 34-year age group, and this could be attributed to the

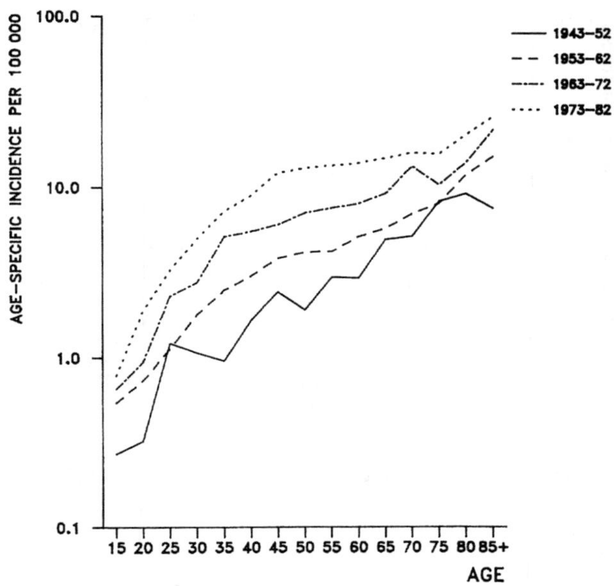

Fig. 6. Age-specific male incidence rates of malignant melanoma of the skin in Denmark, for all sites combined and for successive time periods

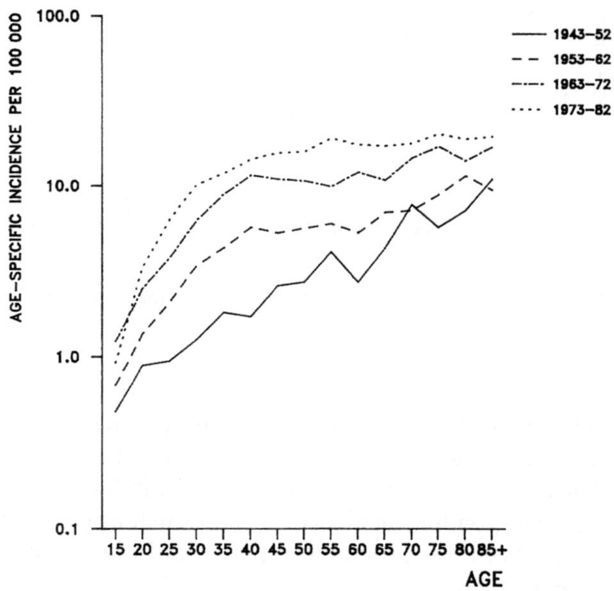

Fig. 7. Age-specific female incidence rates of malignant melanoma of the skin in Denmark, for all sites combined and for successive time periods

pattern seen for the trunk and lower limb. The curves for the upper limb in female patients tend to show a pattern similar to that seen for trunk and lower limb, whereas in male patients the curve for the upper limb does not describe either of the patterns above.

Discussion

Increasing incidence and mortality rates for malignant melanoma of the skin have been reported for the white populations of several developed countries (Jensen and Bolander 1980). These include Denmark, where the rate of increase in the incidence of malignant

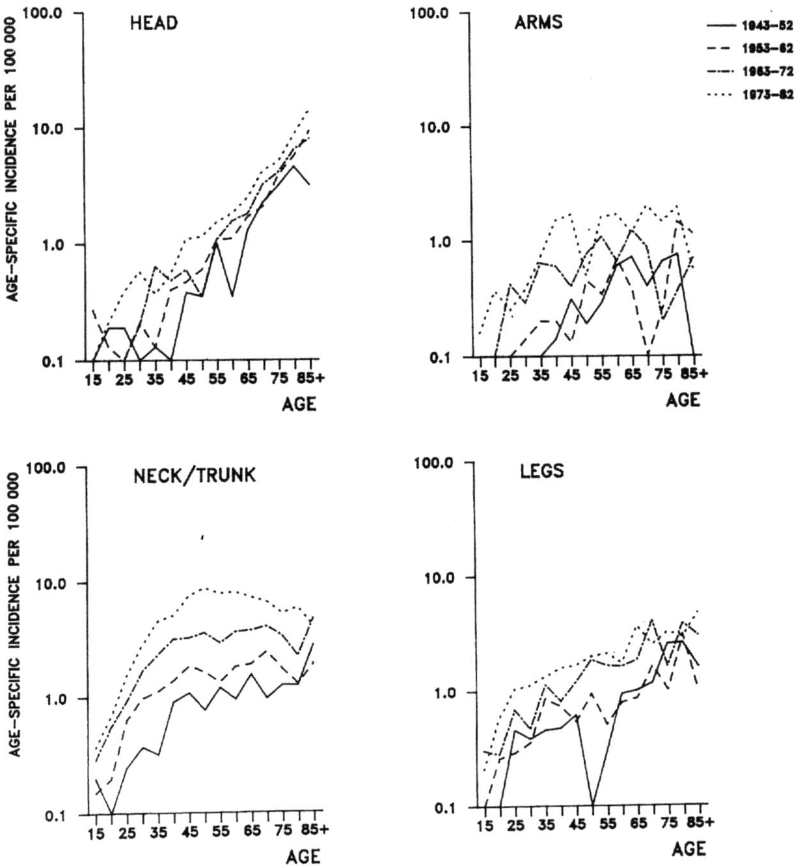

Fig. 8. Age-specific male incidence rates of malignant melanoma of the skin in Denmark, by anatomic site and for successive time periods

melanoma of the skin over the past 40 years has been steeper than for cancer of any other site, including cancer of the lung (Jensen et al. 1985). In cutaneous melanoma the incidence thus rose by factors of 6.1 and 5.1 in female and male subjects, respectively, while the corresponding incidence rate ratios in lung cancer were 5.7 and 5.0. The rise in mortality has been less pronounced than that in incidence (Fig. 2); since 1955 mortality rates have doubled.

The possibility must be considered that the observed increase in the incidence of malignant melanoma could be spurious and attributable to improved diagnosis and cancer registration. Changes in histopathological criteria and in registration efficiency, and higher rates of diagnosis would be expected to result in stepwise increments rather than the gradual increase actually observed. It should be noted that the official histopathological criteria for malignant melanoma of the skin have not changed during the 40-year period. In addition, there is a clear relationship between the rates of increase for incidence and mortality over time, with the mortality trend mirroring the incidence trend with a 10-year lag. It appears likely that the true trend is conveyed by the incidence data rather then the mortality trends, which may be influenced by improvements in treatment and survival.

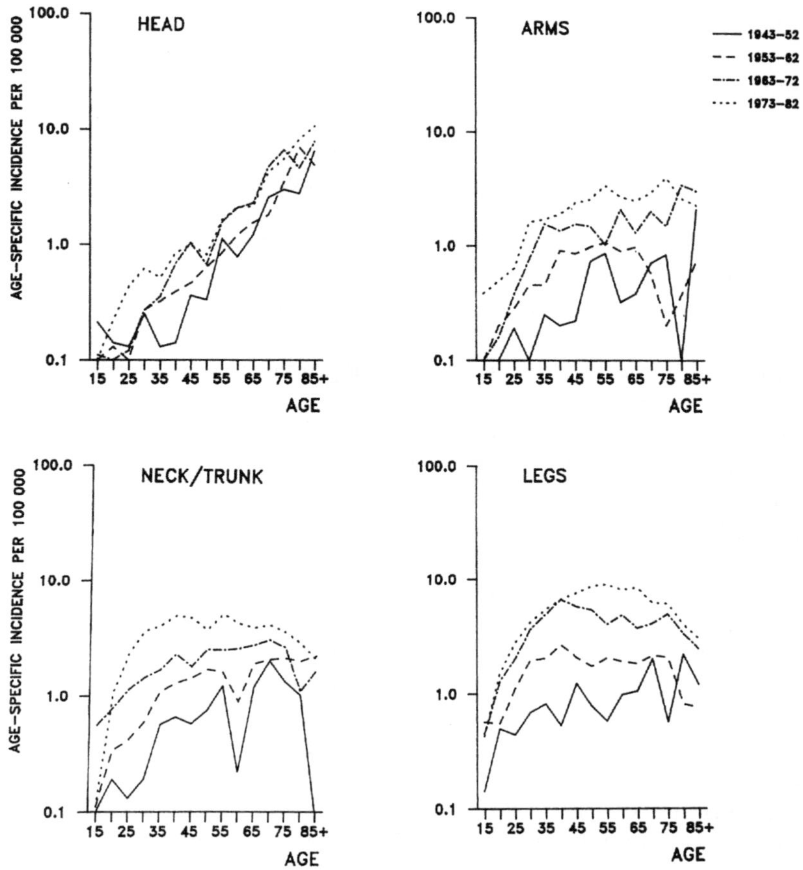

Fig. 9. Age-specific female incidence rates of malignant melanoma of the skin in Denmark by anatomic site and for successive time periods

Furthermore, the increase in incidence has shown specific patterns with regard to sex, age, and anatomic site. Increasing rates are seen for all age groups, but are most prominent among the young, and the increases in incidence have been particularly pronounced for malignant melanoma of the trunk in both sexes and for melanoma of the legs and arms in women, whereas the incidence of malignant melanoma of the head has changed very little. Comparable increases for the same anatomic sites have been reported from other countries (Elwood and Lee 1975; Magnus 1973; Teppo et al. 1978).

The five- to sixfold increase in incidence rates must reflect a substantial increase in exposure to one or more important risk factors. The lack of a levelling of the increase at present may indicate that the rise in risk factor exposure has not yet reached a maximum. The changes have involved both male and female rates, although the rise in incidence rates was most pronounced in women during the decade 1955–1965.

In parallel with the increase in incidence several features of melanoma have changed. Examination of the age-specific incidence curves for four successive 10-year periods reveals that the relative increase in incidence rates is smaller at both ends of the age scale than in between (age groups 20–64 years). Furthermore, the curves show that relatively more young persons develop skin melanoma today than in the 1940s. This change is especially pronounced for female patients. Exposure in an early period of life may therefore be particularly relevant in the etiology of malignant melanoma. Another prominent feature is the difference in trends for the various anatomic sites, which differ for male and female patients. Thus the age-specific male incidence of melanomas on the trunk has hitherto been greater than the female incidence, presumably reflecting that exposure of the trunk has been less common in females than in males. The age-specific incidence curves from the last decade reveal, however, that this relationship has changed. Among young people today women have a greater risk of melanomas on the trunk and the legs than men. The excess in the risk of melanoma of the trunk in young women under 35 years of age has to our knowledge not been described previously.

This extraordinary sex/site-linked relationship indicates that focally acting exogenous factors play a major etiological role. Endogenous or more universally acting factors, such as those related to the general improvement of living conditions in the industrialized countries, are unlikely to lead to such variation in incidence trends by subsites. The total pattern points toward UV light as the most important exogenous risk factor, altered sunbathing habits and different clothing styles explaining major changes in exposure to sunlight (Magnus 1973).

The sharp increase in incidence among young and middle-aged, especially female persons either points to an etiological role of exposure in childhood and adolescence or indicates that the latency period from exposure to diagnosis may be relatively short. When the female age-specific incidence curve rises earlier than the male one a possible explanation may be that girls take up intense sunbathing before boys or may be more susceptible than boys around puberty. It is known that the number of moles increases at puberty (Nicholls 1973), and a positive relationship exists between the number of moles and risk of skin melanomas (Holman and Armstrong 1984). An indirect influence resulting from the endogenous secretion of female sex hormones is possible, but whether endogenous and exogenous steroid hormones play a more direct role in the etiology of malignant melanoma is much more doubtful (Adam et al. 1981; Beral et al. 1977).

The rising incidence and mortality will place increasing demands on treatment and rehabilitation facilities. In addition, there will be psychological and social consequences to the individuals affected by this disease. The increasing public health problem will persist until the etiology of malignant melanoma is sufficiently elucidated to allow intervention.

References

Adam SA, Sheaves JK, Wright NH, Mosser G, Harris RW, Vessey MP (1981) A case-control study of the possible association between oral contraceptives and malignant melanoma. Br J Cancer 44: 45-50

Beral V, Ramcharan S, Faris R (1977) Malignant melanoma and oral contraceptive use among women in California. Br J Cancer 36: 804-809

Clemmesen J (1965) Statisitcal studies in the aetiology of malignant neoplasms, vol 2. Acta Pathol Microbiol Scand [Suppl] 174

Crombie IK (1979a) Racial variation in melanoma incidence Br J Cancer 40: 185-193

Crombie IK (1979b) Variation of melanoma incidence with latitude in North America and Europe. Br J Cancer 40: 774-781

Danish Cancer Registry (1982) Incidence of cancer in Denmark 1973-1977. Danish Cancer Society, Copenhagen

Danish Cancer Registry (1983) Cancer incidence in Denmark 1978, 1979, and 1980. Danish Cancer Society, Copenhagen

Elwood JM, Lee JAH (1975) Recent data on the epidemiology of malignant melanoma. Semin Oncol 2: 149-154

Holman CD, Armstrong BK (1984) Pigmentary traits, ethnic origin, benign nevi, and family history as risk factors for cutaneous malignant melanoma. JNCI 72: 257-266

Jensen OM, Bolander AM (1980) Trends in malignant melanoma of the skin. World Health Stat Q 33: 3-26

Jensen OM, Storm HH, Jensen HS (1985) Cancer registration in multiple primary cancers in Denmark 1943-80. Natl Cancer Inst Monogr 68: 245-251

Little JH, Holt J, Davis N (1980) The changing epidemiology of malignant melanoma in Queensland. Med J Aust 1: 66-69

Magnus K (1973) Incidence of malignant melanoma of the skin in Norway 1955-70. Variation in time and space and solar radiation. Cancer 32: 1275-1286

Magnus K (1977) Incidence of malignant melanoma of the skin in the five Nordic countries. Significance of solar radiation. Int J Cancer 20: 447-485

Nicholls EM (1973) Development and elimination of pigmented moles, and the anatomical distribution of primary malignant melanoma. Cancer 32: 191-195

Østerlind A, Jensen OM (1985) Evaluation of the registration of cancer cases in Denmark in 1977. Preliminary evaluation of registration of cancer cases by the Cancer Register and the National Patient Register. Ugeskr laeger

Teppo L, Pakkanen M, Hakulinen T (1978) Sunlight as a risk factor of malignant melanoma of the skin. Cancer 41: 2018-2027

Waterhouse J, Muir C, Correa P, Powell J (1976) Cancer incidence in five continents, vol 3. IARC, Lyons (Scientific publications, no. 42)

Waterhouse J, Muir C, Shanmugartnam K, Powell J (1982) Cancer incidence in five continents, vol 4. IARC, Lyons (Scientific publications, no. 42)

*The Causes of Malignant Melanoma: Results from the West Australian Lions Melanoma Research Project**, **

C. D. J. Holman, B. K. Armstrong, P. J. Heenan, J. B. Blackwell, F. J. Cumming, D. R. English, S. Holland, G. R. H. Kelsall, L. R. Matz, I. L. Rouse, A. Singh, R. E. J. Ten Seldam, J. D. Watt, and Z. Xu

Epidemiology Branch, Health Department of Western Australia, 60 Beaufort Street, Perth 6000, Australia

Introduction

In Australia malignant melanoma ranks forth among cancers as a cause of morbidity and premature death (Armstrong 1985). For this reason, and because the State of Western Australia has one of the highest incidence rates of melanoma in the world (Holman et al. 1980), we undertook a multidisciplinary research program embracing the epidemiology, histopathology, and clinical management of melanoma. A major component of our research was a population-based case-control study in which constitutional traits, sunlight exposure, hormones, diet and other possible causal factors were evaluated. We have already published several reports of the results relating to particular subject areas (Holman and Armstrong 1983, 1984 a, b; Holman et al. 1984 b, 1985; English et al. 1985). In this report we aim to bring together in summary form the key results of the project to date and to present new data on diet and other factors.

Methods

Detailed accounts of the materials and methods can be found in the publications cited above. What follows is a brief summary of the study design and methods of analysis.

The case series comprised 511 patients with histologically proven preinvasive or invasive melanoma of the skin. They represented 76% of a total of 670 newly incident eligible cases less than 80 years of age and resident in accessible regions of Western Australia during a period of 675 days beginning 1 January 1980. Thirteen percent of eligible cases were excluded from interview for medical reasons, and durther 11% were either untraceable or uncooperative. A panel of six pathologists classified sections from the tumours of all but 14 of the 511 patients, according to whether the histological type of melanoma was Hutch-

* Supported by the Lions Club of Western Australia and the Cancer Foundation of Western Australia. CDJH was supported by a Medical Postgraduate Research Scholarship of the National Health and Medical Research Council of Australia

** *Abbreviations: HMF,* Hutchinson's melanotic freckle; *SSM,* superficial spreading melanoma; *NM,* nodular melanoma; *UCM,* unclassified melanoma; *CMT,* cutaneous microtopography; *UVR,* ultraviolet radiation; *ROEP,* Recreational outdoor exposure proportion; *OCP,* oral contraceptive preparations

Recent Results in Cancer Research. Vol 102

inson's melanotic freckle (HMF), superficial spreading melanoma (SSM), unclassifiable melanoma (UCM), or nodular melanoma (NM) (McGovern et al. 1973). Clinical details, including information on primary site, was obtained from the general practitioners and surgeons who attended the patients.

Control subjects were randomly selected from the Australian Commonwealth Electoral Roll and were matched to the cases for sex, 5-year birth period, and electoral subdivision. For 10 cases aged less than 18 years matched controls were selected from the student rolls of public schools. The final series of 511 controls arose from 824 selections of potential subjects, many of whom could not be traced or refused to take part. Overall, 69% of potential controls approached were interviewed, compared with 90% of melanoma patients who were approached. The methods of contacting potential participants and soliciting their cooperation were identical for patients and controls.

Subjects were interviewed in their homes or occasionally at their workplaces by trained nurse interviewers who, to the extent possible, were blind as to which subjects were cases and which were controls. The following information and specimens were collected: (a) A highly structured questionnaire regarding constitutional and genetic factors, history of sun exposure, hormone use, diet, and several other factors; (b) a 24-h dietary record; (c) objective records of skin, eye, and hair colour; weight; height; amount of body hair; number of raised naevi on the arms; and extent of actinic skin damage measured by cutaneous microtopography; and (d) a voluntary venous blood sample for retinol and cholesterol assays.

The methods of analysis were those described by Breslow and Day (1980) for matched case-control studies. Odds ratios were calculated by conditional maximum likelihood estimation. Conditional logistic regression analysis of the simultaneous effects of two or more factors was performed by a FORTRAN package (Thomas 1980). Four controls with a past history of melanoma were excluded from analysis, together with their corresponding cases.

It was necessary to control for bias due to several types of confounding in this study. Positive confounding occurred between the different constitutional traits typical of fair-skinned individuals, between unfavourable skin response to sunlight and history of sunburn as well as use of sunscreens, and between late age of arrival of migrants to Australia and participation in high sun exposure activities. Negative confounding was apparent between unfavourable skin response and high sun exposure activities, and between unfavourable skin response and tendency to wear scant clothing. In each instance the relevant analyses were controlled for these effects by inclusion of the confounding variables in the logistic regression models.

Where necessary, additional information on the methods is included with the results.

Results

Pigmentary Traits

The following factors indicative of external body pigmentation and skin response to sunlight exposure were recorded: Chronic skin reaction to sunlight (i.e., ability to tan), acute skin reaction to sunlight (i.e., tendency to burn), hair colour, eye colour, and skin colour measured at the left upper inner arm, left shoulder tip, and dorsum of the left hand. Overall melanoma risk was strongly related to each of these factors, with the exception of skin colour of the shoulder tip and dorsum of hand. The rates of melanoma were highest in

Table 1. Relationship of histological types of malignant melanoma to chronic skin reaction to sunlight

Histological type		Chronic skin reaction to sunlight				P value of trend
		Deep tan	Moderate tan	Mild tan	No tan	
HMF:	OR	1.0	2.3	5.3	10.0	
	95% CI		1.1–5.0	1.9–14.5	1.0–103.0	<0.001
SSM:	OR	1.0	1.3	1.8	2.8	
	95% CI		0.9–1.9	1.1–2.8	1.2–6.6	0.002
UCM	OR	1.0	1.1	2.6	2.5	
	95% CI		0.5–2.2	1.0–6.7	0.5–11.9	0.057
NM:	OR	1.0	1.8	2.5[a]		
	95% CI		0.7–4.5	0.8–7.8		0.083

[a] Mild tan and no tan were combined

persons with poor tanning ability, a tendency to develop severe sunburn, fair or red hair colour, blue or green eye colour, and very pale baseline skin colour as measured at the inner upper arm (Holman and Armstrong 1984a). However, when these variables were included simultaneously in a logistic regression model, only chronic and acute skin reactions to sunlight and hair colour appeared to have independent effects.

Chronic skin reaction to sunlight was the strongest risk indicator out of those related to pigmentary traits. The relationship of each histologic type of melanoma to chronic reaction to sunlight is shown in Table 1. HMF had the strongest association, whereas the empirical strengths of the association with poor tanning ability were similar among the other three histological types.

Ethnic Origin

The four grandparents of each subject were classified according to wheterh they were Celtic (Irish, Scottish or Welsh), English, Australian (probably Celtic or English), southern European (mainly Italian, Yugoslav and Greek), northern European, African, or Asian. The relationships of all melanomas combined to possession of two or more grandparents belonging to each ethnic group were examined, controlling for confounding effects of age on arrival in Australia (Holman and Armstrong 1984a). Reduced rates of melanoma were observed in persons having two or more southern European grandparents (OR=0.4; 95% CI=0.2–0.9), and also in those with two or more grandparents of northern European (OR=0.6; 95% CI=0.3–1.0) or Asian or African origin (OR=0.4; 95% CI= <0.1–3.3).

Contrary to the expected result, persons with two or more Celtic grandparents did not have a particularly high odds ratio in this study (OR=1.2; 95% CI 0.8–1.7).

Family History of Melanoma

A family history of melanoma was reported by 15% of patients and 6% of controls. In relation to the number of affected blood relatives, odds ratios for all melanomas combined, with no affected blood relatives as the reference category, were 2.3 (1.4–3.5) in persons

Table 2. Relationship of histological types of malignant melanoma to presence of raised naevi on the arms and history of excision of benign moles

Histological type	Presence of raised naevi on the arms		History of excision of benign moles	
	OR	95% CI	OR	95% CI
HMF	1.5	0.7–3.3	1.5	0.6–4.0
SSM	3.0	2.0–4.6	2.4	1.3–4.3
UCM	1.6	0.8–3.2	1.8	0.6–5.6
NM	3.0	1.1–8.4	2.0	0.6–6.7

with one affected blood relative and 5.0 (1.4–17.3) in those with two or more affected blood relatives. Having one or more affected relatives by marriage, including a spouse with melanoma, did not appear to confer any excess risk (OR = 1.0; 95% CI = 0.5–2.0). Empirically, HMF had the strongest association with family history, whereas the association was of intermediate strength for SSM and NM (Holman and Armstrong 1984a).

Benign Naevi

The number of raised naevi counted on both arms below the level of the axillae was a very strong risk indicator in this study. Because nonpalpable naevi were excluded from the count to avoid confusion with freckles, the enumeration procedure may have been biased in favour of compound and intradermal naevi rather than junctional naevi. Despite this limitation and the exclusion from the count of naevi occurring on skin other than that of the arms, the measure obtained was considered to provide a surrogate for the number of naevi on the body with a potential for malignant change at an earlier time of life.

Compared with persons having no naevi on the arms, there was an increasing gradient in odds ratios, ranging from 2.0 for one to four naevi to 11.3 in persons with ten or more naevi. Results for each histological type pertaining to presence of raised naevi on the arms, and also history of surgical excision of benign moles, are shown in Table 2. Empirically and statistically the association was strongest for SSM and weakest for HMF (Holman and Armstrong 1984a).

Cutaneous Microtopography

Patients and controls interviewed in the Perth metropolitan area (76% of all pairs) underwent measurement of the extent of actinic skin damage by CMT (Holman and Armstrong 1984b). This technique involved taking a silicone rubber impression of the skin texture on the back of the hand and later grading it under a low-power microscope according to the extent of changes considered to reflect prolonged sunlight exposure (Beagley and Gibson 1980). Evidence of the validity of CMT as an indicator of accumulated sun exposure has been reported (Holman et al. 1984a).

The results (Table 3) showed that HMF had the strongest apparent association with actinic skin damage. No case of HMF had a microtopograph graded less than 4, necessitat-

Table 3. Relationships of histological types of malignant melanoma to actinic skin damage graded by cutaneous microtopography

Histological type		CMT grade				*P* value of trend
		1-3	4	5	6	
HMF:	OR	1.0[a]		4.0	4.4	
	95% CI			0.9-17.7	1.2-15.7	0.048
SSM:	OR	1.0	1.5	2.2	2.6	
	95% CI		0.8-2.9	1.0-4.9	1.1-6.1	0.021
UCM:	OR	1.0	2.7	0.6	1.2	
	95% CI		0.7-10.4	0.2-2.2	0.3-4.4	0.652
NM:	OR	1.0	0.6	0.9	5.2	
	95% CI		0.1-5.6	0.1-14.1	0.3-98.7	0.092

[a] Grades 1-3 and 4 were combined

ing the inclusion of grade 4 in the baseline category in Table 3. For SSM a less pronounced association with CMT was seen, although statistically the association was accompanied by a *p* value of 0.021. There was no evidence of a consistent association of CMT grade with UCM.

History of Nonmelanotic Skin Cancer

A past history of a skin cancer, other than a malignant mole, which had been treated by surgery or radiotherapy was a strong risk factor for all types of melanoma, particularly HMF (Holman and Armstrong 1984b). Compared with persons with no history of nonmelanotic skin cancer, the odds ratios were 5.2 (1.7-18.0) for HMF, 3.3 (1.3-9.3) for SSM, 3.0 (1.0-9.4) for UCM, and 5.0 (0.6-113.1) for NM.

Age on Arrival and Duration of Residence in Australia

In all, 23% of subjects in the study were migrants, mostly from the British Isles. For all types of melanoma combined, there was evidence that the incidence rate increased with longer duration of residence in Australia, and with earlier age on first arrival. A stepped logistic regression analysis was performed to determine whether living in Australia at an early age, or simply the total number of years lived in Australia, was the more important factor. The largest contribution to goodness of fit was made by age on arrival in Australia, with duration of residence having no residual effect (Holman and Armstrong 1984b).

For SSM, the effect of age on arrival appeared specific to certain age groups (Table 4). The results, controlled for potential confounding with ethnic origin, suggested that the incidence rate of SSM in migrants arriving before the age of 10 years was near to or greater than that in the native-born population (ages 0-4, OR = 1.2; ages 5-9, OR = 1.6). Migrants arriving at ages 10-14 years had an odds ratio of 0.7, and a further reduction was seen in migrants arriving at 15-19 years of age (OR = 0.2). However, arrival at ages later than 19 years appeared to give no additional protective effect, the incidence rate in late-arriving

Table 4. Relationships of histological types of malignant melanoma to mean annual hours of bright sunlight, with pseudo-restriction to native-born Australians

Histological type		Migrants	Native-born Australians			
			Mean annual hours of bright sunlight			*P* value of trend
			<2600	2600-2799	2800^+	
HMF:	OR	0.2	1.0	1.5	3.8	
	95% CI	0.1-0.7		0.6-4.2	0.5-26.4	0.101
SSM:	OR	0.4	1.0	1.2	2.1	
	95% CI	0.3-0.7		0.7-2.0	0.9-5.0	0.020
UCM:	OR	0.9	1.0	0.8	1.4	
	95% CI	0.4-1.9		0.3-1.8	0.5-4.3	0.922
NM:	OR	0.1	1.0	0.3	0.3	
	95% CI	0.02-0.5		0.04-2.9	0.04-2.6	0.193

migrants stabilizing at around one-quarter to one-third of the native-born rate (ages 20-24 and 25-29, OR = 0.2; ages 30+, OR = 0.4; P for trend <0.001).

Within the control subjects of predominantly Celtic or English ancestry, it was observed that controls born in Australia or first arriving before the age of 10 years had more raised naevi on the arms than controls arriving at or after the age of 10 years ($P=0.009$). Possibly sun exposure in childhood is a factor in the production of benign naevi, which have their strongest relationship with SSM, probably as precursor lesions.

Annual Hours of Bright Sunlight

From a detailed residential history and use of a climatology map (Landsberg 1966), the annual hours of bright sunshine at residential locations were averaged over a subject's lifetime and over specific periods of life (Holman and Armstrong 1984b). Table 4 shows the relationship between the different histological types of melanoma and mean annual hours of bright sunshine averaged over the whole of life. Migrants to Australia were removed from the main body of the analysis by placing them in a special category for comparison with native-born Australians with the lowest residential sunlight exposure. Except for UCM, migrants consistently had a reduced incidence rate of each histological type. For HMF and SSM there were gradients of increasing odds ratios with greater numbers of mean annual hours of bright sunshine within the group of native-born Australians. Empirically, the gradient was strongest for HMF. UCM and NM were not positively associated with mean annual hours of bright sunshine.

The effects of residential exposure to high levels of sunlight at ages 0-9, 10-24, 25-39, and 40 or more years were examined. High exposure (2800 annual hours or more of bright sunlight) at ages 10-24 years appeared to be a strong risk factor for SSM when compared with having consistently low to moderate residential exposure throughout life (OR = 11.3; 95% CI = 1.4-91.1). High exposure at ages 25-39 years also was associated with an increased rate of SSM (OR = 3.4; 95% CI = 1.4-8.2), whereas high exposure at ages 0-9 years and at 40 years or more seemed to have no effect. Little could be made of the results for other histological types.

Table 5. Relationship of histological types of malignant melanoma to recreational outdoor exposure proportion in summer at ages 10–24 years, controlled for potential confounders[a]

Histological type		Recreational outdoor exposure proportion in summer at ages 10–24 years (%)				P value of trend
		0–29	30–39	40–59	60+	
HMF:	OR	1.0	1.0	1.9	0.8	
	95% CI		0.3–3.8	0.5–7.4	0.2–2.9	0.943
SSM:	OR	1.0	1.2	1.7	1.6	
	95% CI		0.6–2.3	0.9–3.1	0.9–2.8	0.148
UCM:	OR	1.0	1.3	0.8	0.8	
	95% CI		0.4–4.1	0.3–2.4	0.3–2.2	0.544
NM:	OR	1.0	1.8	0.4	3.5	
	95% CI		0.2–13.6	0.1–2.5	0.7–18.4	0.258

[a] Chronic and acute skin reaction to sunlight, hair colour, ethnic origin, and age on arrival in Australia

Occupational and Recreational Outdoor Exposure

Estimates of the mean hours per week spent outdoors were derived for each subject based on detailed occupational and recreational histories. Separate estimates were made for summer and winter, for outdoor exposure during work and leisure, and for specific periods of life as well as total working life. With the exception of HMF, all histological types appeared inversely associated with total outdoor exposure (i.e., the sum of work and leisure exposures). For SSM and NM the inverse association with total outdoor exposure appeared strongest at ages 10–24 years. Compared with persons having uniformly low outdoor exposure (fewer than 23 h per week) in all periods of working life, those with high outdoor exposure at ages 10–24 years had an adjusted odds ratio of 0.4 (0.2–1.0) for SSM and 0.1 (0.01–1.3) for NM (Holman et al. 1985).

To evaluate the effects of intermittency of outdoor exposure, we derived a "recreational outdoor exposure proportion" (ROEP), which expressed recreational outdoor exposure as a proportion of total outdoor exposure in summer. Table 5 shows the relationships of histological types to ROEP based on recreational and total outdoor exposure at ages 10–24 years. Although SSM was associated with ROEP at ages 10–24 the relationship was weak and may have arisen by chance.

Water Sports and Sunbathing

The popularity of water sports and sunbathing as recreational pastimes in Western Australia raises the possibility that they might be involved in the development of melanoma. especially SSM. The relevant results are in Table 6.

SSM was associated with frequent participation in boating and fishing, but was only very weakly associated with swimming or sunbathing. For sunbathing at ages 15–24 years the evidence was stronger when the analysis was confined to SSM occurring on the trunk (Table 6). Frequency of sunbathing was also examined within the 10 years before diagnosis of the case, but the strengths of association were weak compared with SSM of the trunk

Table 6. Relationship of superficial spreading melanoma to frequency of participation in aquatic activities and sunbathing in summer, controlled for potential confounders[a]

Outdoor activity		Frequency of participation in summer aquatic activities and sunbathing			*P* value of trend
		Never	Less than once/week	Once or more/week	
Boating:	OR	1.0	1.1	2.4	
	95% CI		0.5-2.1	1.1-5.4	0.043
Fishing:	OR	1.0	1.0	2.7	
	95% CI		0.6-1.7	1.2-6.4	0.071
Swimming:	OR	1.0	1.3	1.1	
	95% CI		0.8-2.2	0.7-1.8	0.663
Sunbathing, ages 15-24 years					
All SSM:	OR	1.0	1.3	1.3	
	95% CI		0.8-2.0	0.8-2.2	0.263
SSM on trunk:	OR	1.0	1.2	2.6	
	95% CI		0.5-2.8	1.0-6.2	0.044

[a] Chronic and acute skin reaction to sunlight, hair colour, ethnic origin, and age an arrival in Australia

and sunbathing at ages 10-24 years. Frequencies of boating, fishing, and swimming in different periods of life were not recorded (Holman et al. 1985).

Clothing Habits

Habits of dress during outdoor work were assessed at the time of recording occupational history. Except for SSM, oods ratios were higher for persons in whom the site of the melanoma had been sometimes exposed rather than usually exposed or usually covered (Holman et al. 1985). There was, however, a linear association of SSM with body site exposure during outdoor work, which was strongest for SSM occurring on the trunk. Compared with persons who usually covered their trunk, adjusted odds ratios for SSM of the trunk were 2.9 (1.0-85.) in those sometimes exposed and 6.0 (0.4-112.1) in those who were usually exposed while working outdoors (*P* for trend = 0.032).

The type of bathing suit worn by women at the beach in summer was apparently a strong determinant of both SSM and other histological types of melanoma of the trunk. The adjusted odds ratio for all melanomas of the trunk was estimated at 13.0 (2.0-83.9) in women who wore a bikini or bathed nude at ages 15-24 years, compared with those who wore a one-piece swimsuit with a high backline. Women wearing a swimsuit with a low backline had an intermediate odds ratio of 4.0 (0.6-25.2; *P* for trend = 0.005). A similar but weaker result was observed for type of bathing suit worn by women within 10 years before diagnosis in the case (Holman et al. 1985).

Sunlamps

Past use of artificial sunlamps was recorded, but only 9% of subjects had used them. The unadjusted odds ratio relating all melanomas to having ever used a sunlamp was 1.1 (0.6–1.8). Results for the histological types were of little value owing to wide confidence intervals (Holman 1982).

Body Hair

We previously formed an hypothesis that differences between the sexes in the site distribution of melanoma, and specifically the greater proportion of lower limb melanomas in women, might be explained by different body hair distributions (Holman and Armstrong 1982). To test this hypothesis photographs of forearm hair and calf hair were taken from subjects interviewed in the Perth metropolitan area, and graded according to the extent of body hair on a three-step scale (Holman 1982). The relationships of all melanomas and those occurring on the lower and upper limbs to extent of calf and forearm hair were examined. Because of the tendency for persons of dark complexion to have more abundant body hair than fair persons, the analyses were controlled for confounding by hair colour. No evidence of any inverse association was observed. For melanoma of the lower limb, compared with persons having abundant calf hair, adjusted odds ratios were 1.1 (0.3–4.4) in those with sparse calf hair and 0.9 (0.3–2.9) in those with no hair on their calves (P for trend = 0.978).

Sunburn

Histories of sunburn of varying degrees of severity were obtained during the interviews, and 76% of subjects reported a history of peeling sunburn. Painful sunburn lasting 2 or more days was reported by 64%, and 36% of subjects stated that they had suffered from

Table 7. Relationship of histological types of malignant melanoma to highest severity of past sunburn, controlled for potential confounders[a]

Histological type		Highest severity of past sunburn				P value of trend
		No sunburn	Peeling sunburn	Painful sunburn	Blistering sunburn	
HMF:	OR	1.0	0.6	2.4	2.8	
	95% CI		0.2–2.6	0.6–9.7	0.7–10.4	0.059
SSM:	OR	1.0	0.8	0.6	1.0	
	95%CI		0.4–1.7	0.3–1.1	0.6–2.0	0.714
UCM:	OR	1.0	0.8	1.4	1.2	
	95% CI		0.2–2.6	0.5–4.0	0.5–2.9	0.681
NM:	OR 95% CI	1.0	0.5	0.2	0.05	
			0.1–4.8	0.03–1.4	0.01–0.6	0.010

[a] Chronic and acute skin reaction to sunlight, hair colour, ethnic origin, and age on arrival in Australia

sunburn with blisters. It appeared, therefore, that the ranking of severity of sunburn in this study was probably peeling sunburn, painful sunburn, blistering sunburn.

In Table 7 odds ratios for melanoma of different histological types are given in relation to highest severity of past sunburn. Before control for confounding, the odds ratios had been higher due to association of sunburn with fair skin type and early age on arrival in Australia. Nevertheless, after control there was some evidence that HMF was related to severe sunburn (*P* for trend = 0.059). For NM severe sunburn appeared to be protective. SSM and UCM were unrelated to sunburn history after confounding was controlled Holman et al. 1985).

Sunscreens

Frequency and duration of sunscreen use were studied but appeared to have little effect on the rates of all melanomas combined or of any particular histological type. Compared with persons who never used sunscreens (42% of those exposing skin other than the face or arms), adjusted odds ratios for all melanomas were 1.1 (0.7–1.6) for duration of use less than 10 years, and 1.2 (0.8–1.7) in persons using sunscreens for 10 years or more (*P* for trend = 0.479). It should be noted, however, that effective sunscreening agents were not widely available in Australia at the time when most subjects in the study were in early adulthood (Holman et al. 1985).

Fluorescent Lighting

Following the publication of another study in which melanoma was found to be associated with exposure to fluorescent lighting at work (Beral et al. 1982), 337 of our cases and 349 controls were reinterviewed in 1983 regarding fluorescent light exposure (English et al. 1985). The incidence of all melanomas was not associated with rate of exposure or cumulative exposure to all fluorescent lights or exposure to only those without diffusers. With a cumulative exposure of less than 10000 h as the baseline, odds ratios for all melanomas were 0.8 (0.5–1.2) for 10000–19999 h of exposure, 1.0 (0.6–1.5) for 20000–34999 h and 1.2 (0.8–1.9) for cumulative exposure of 35000 h or more (*P* for trend = 0.27).

When the histological types and different body sites were examined separately, only the incidence rate of UCM increased with increasing duration of exposure (*P* for trend = 0.02). This association was weaker and the *P* value higher (0.11) when exposure only in residential rooms and offices, where light fittings were closer to the subjects, was considered (English et al. 1985).

Ionizing Radiation

By use of interview data on occupations, and a linkage system for the study of occupational carcinogenesis developed by Hoar et al. (1980), it was estimated that 11% of male cases and 10% of controls had been exposed to ionizing radiation at some time during working life. Odds ratios for histological types suggested an association of HMF with occupational exposure to ionizing radiation (OR = 2.7; 95% CI = 1.0–6.9). For NM, ionizing radiation exposure at work appeared to be protective, based on ten discordant case-control pairs, each with an exposed control (*P* = 0.004). Odds ratios for SSM and UCM were 1.6 (0.8–3.0) and 0.2 (0.02–1.4), respectively.

Therapeutic exposure to ionizing radiation was also examined (Holman 1982). A history of radiotherapy for conditions other than skin cancer was associated with SSM (OR=3.0; 95% CI=1.0-9.4). Other odds ratios were 1.5 (0.4-6.3) for HMF, 0.7 (0.2-5.5) for UCM and 0.4 (0.1-1.8) for NM.

Reproductive Factors

In the 276 female case-control pairs we examined the effects of age at menarche, duration of menstrual life in those who were postmenopausal, number of pregnancies of 20 or more weeks' duration, and degree of obesity assessed by Quetelet's index. Obesity was studied because of its known association with plasma estrogen levels especially in postmenopausal women. Neither all melanomas combined nor any histological type was associated with any of these factors (Holman et al. 1984b).

Oral Contraceptive Preparations

Past or present use of OCPs was reported by 53% of female subjects. Odds ratios relating total duration of use to histological types of melanoma are given in Table 8. While the results were not inconsistent with an elevation of the rates of HMF and SSM in women who had used OCP for 2 or more years, the estimated effects were readily explained by chance and the evidence of linear dose response was weak. For ever-use of OCP an odds ratio of 1.0 (0.6-1.6) was observed for all melanomas, whereas for SSM the odds ratio was 1.1 (0.6-2.2).

The association of melanoma subtypes with OCP use was examined within intervals of 10 or more years, 5-9 years, and less than 5 years before diagnosis of the case. There was little empirical evidence of an effect of OCP use in any of the time periods studied (Holman et al. 1984b).

Table 8. Relationships of histological types of malignant melanoma in women to duration of use of oral contraceptive preparations

Histological type		Duration of OCP use (years)				*P* value of trend
		Never	<2	2-4	5+	
HMF:	OR	1.0	0.3	4.6[a]		
	95% CI		0.03-2.6	0.5-40.4		0.145
SSM:	OR	1.0	0.8	1.7	1.5	
	95% CI		0.4-1.7	0.7-3.9	0.7-3.2	0.177
UCM:	OR	1.0	0.6	0.7	0.8	
	95% CI		0.1-2.2	0.2-2.3	0.2-2.8	0.802
NM:	OR	1.0		0.3[b]		
	95% CI			0.02-3.6		0.617

[a] 2-4 years and 5+ years were combined
[b] Ever-use of OCP

Other Oestrogenic Preparations

Of the female subjects, 14% had taken hormone tablets or injections containing an oestrogen but no progestagen at some time. The relationship of each histological type to duration of oestrogen use was examined; only for SSM was there borderline evidence of linear dose response. Compared with women who had never taken unopposed oestrogen preparations, odds ratios for SSM were 1.7 (0.7-4.1) for up to 1 year's duration of use and 2.3 (0.8-6.2) for more than 1 year of use (P for trend = 0.082).

Diet

Nutritional factors were assessed in the interview by a food frequency questionnaire and by a 24-h dietary record completed the day before the interview took place. According to the 24-h diet records there was essentially no difference between total cases and controls in mean intakes of protein, fat, carbohydrate, alcohol, retinol, beta carotene, acorbic acid, riboflavin, thiamine, niacin, calcium, phosphorus, iron, sodium, and potassium (Holman 1982). The same conclusion was reached for each histological type, except that NM patients had higher intakes of protein and fat than matched controls. The mean daily protein intake was 89 g in NM cases, compared with 73 g in controls ($P = 0.004$), and mean daily fat consumptions were 107 g and 89 g in NM cases and controls, respectively ($P = 0.016$).

Food items chosen for inclusion in the food frequency questionnaire were those high in animal fat or cholesterol; those containing high levels of retinoids, beta carotene or ascorbic acid; vegetables of the *Brassicaceae* family; barbecued or smoked foods; and polyunsaturated margarine. These items were chosen because of their suspected or possible role as causal or protective factors in cancer development. Results pertaining to margarine and foods high in vitamin A content are described below. There was no evidence of association of any of the remainder of foods with melanomas of the HMF, SSM, or UCM types. For NM there was some evidence of association with certain meats shown in Table 9. Also described in Table 9 are the associations of NM with protein and fat measured by the 24-h dietary record.

Polyunsaturated Fats

Polyunsaturated fats have been hypothesized to be a cause of malanoma (Mackie et al. 1980). From the food frequency questionnaire we found no evidence of association of melanoma with frequency of margarine consumption. Compared with those taking margarine less than once per month, melanoma odds ratios were 1.0 (0.6-1.9) for margarine consumption once or more per month but less than once per day, 1.2 (0.8-1.9) for once per day consumption, and 1.0 (0.7-1.4) for margarine consumption twice or more per day (P for trend = 0.998).

We also collected information on the type of cooking oil or fat used in the preparation of fried foods. Again, no evidence of a relationship was found. Odds ratios for all melanomas, with animal fat as the reference category, were 1.2 (0.7-1.8) in those using moderately unsaturated oils and 0.9 (0.6-1.2) for use of highly unsaturated oils. Neither consumption of margarine nor type of cooking oil or fat was related to any histological type of melanoma (Holman 1982).

Table 9. Relationships of nodular malenoma to level of consumption of protein, fat, and various meats

Nutrient or food item	Consumption level Low ⟵			⟶ High	*P* value of trend
Protein:[a]					
OR	1.0	2.0	4.8	7.8	
95% CI		0.4–10.5	0.6–36.1	1.1–53.7	0.011
Fat:[a]					
OR	1.0	2.0	1.4	3.7	
95% CI		0.5–7.7	0.3–6.8	0.9–15.0	0.072
Beef:[b]					
OR	1.0	0.6	0.5		
95% CI		0.1–2.6	0.1–1.9		0.316
Veal or lamb:[b]					
OR	1.0	0.8	1.1	2.1	
95% CI		0.3–2.6	0.4–2.7	0.4–9.8	0.467
Pork, bacon or lamb:[b]					
OR	1.0	1.8	2.2	2.7	
95% CI		0.6–5.9	0.9–5.7	0.8–9.5	0.045
Poultry:[b]					
OR	1.0	5.2	3.5	5.3	
95% CI		1.0–26.2	0.7–18.0	0.8–35.1	0.380

[a] Measured by a 24-h dietary record
[b] Measured by a food frequency questionnaire

Serum Retinol and Dietary Beta Carotene

There was little difference between cases and controls in mean daily intakes of retinol or beta carotene assessed by the 24-h dietary records (Holman 1982). Examination of food frequency results relating to carrots, pumpkin, and silverbeet (all high in beta carotene) also revealed no evidence of effect. Consumption of liver, a concentrated source of retinoids, more than once per month appeared to afford borderline protection with an odds ratio for all melanomas of 0.7 (0.6–1.0). However, in persons who took vitamin A supplements there was a modest elevation in risk (OR = 1.4: 95% CI = 0.9–2.3). The conclusion derived from the balance of these data was that the results did not support an effect on melanoma incidence by dietary beta carotene or retinoids.

Measurement of serum retinol was introduced late in the study. Blood samples were taken and analysed from 141 cases and 140 controls. Mean serum levels of retinol were 53.9 mg/l in cases and 56.4 mg/l in controls ($P = 0.469$). When retinol concentrations were divided by tertiles (<44, 44–58 and 59+ mg/litre), the odds ratios for all melanomas comparing the middle and upper tertiles with the lower tertile were 1.0 (0.5–1.8) and 0.6 (0.3–1.1), respectively (P for trend = 0.623).

Table 10. Relationships of histological types of malignant melanoma to current level of alcohol consumption

Histological type		Current level of alcohol intake (kg/year)				*P* value of trend
		None	1-2	3-9	10+	
HMF:	OR	1.0	1.5	1.2	1.4	
	95% CI		0.6-3.7	0.5-3.1	0.5-3.6	0.846
SSM:	OR	1.0	0.7	1.2	1.0	
	95% CI		0.4-1.2	0.7-1.9	0.6-1.7	0.335
UCM:	OR	1.0	1.8	2.9	2.5	
	95% CI		0.8-4.3	1.2-7.1	1.0-6.3	0.068
NM:	OR	1.0	1.6	1.9	1.7	
	95% CI		0.4-6.2	0.5-7.2	0.4-6.9	0.650

Alcohol

Levels of intake of alcoholic beverages were recorded in the interview. Separate assessments were made for beer, wine and spirits. An estimate of current total alcohol intake in kilograms per year was calculated as the sum of intakes of beer, wine, and spirits. each weighted by the average alcohol content of common Western Australian beverages (beer 0.04 g/ml; wine 0.12 g/ml; spirits 0.5 g/ml).

The relationships of histological types of melanoma to current alcohol consumption level are shown in Table 10. Only for UCM was there reasonable evidence of an increased incidence rate in those consuming more than 3 kg alcohol per year. When the three types of alcoholic beverage were examined separately, the rate of UCM increased with increasing current consumption of beer, wine, and spirits. The association of UCM with alcohol was observed only in current drinkers. Past drinkers of each type of beverage had on odds ratio less than unity (Holman 1982).

Hair Dyes

Subjects were asked the number of times they had used permanent and nonpermanent (i.e., semipermanent and temporary) hair dyes. There was little evidence of any association of melanoma with use of permanent hair dyes (Holman and Armstrong 1983). For nonpermanent dyes there appeared to be a specific relationship between frequency of dye use and HMF (see Table 11). Further examination of the data showed that the association did not apply to head and neck melanoma other than HMF, but did apply to HMF occurring at other body sites.

Lower Limb Shaving and Depilation

Trauma through shaving or depilation has been suggested as an explanation for the higher rate of melanoma of the lower limb in women than in men (Lee and Merrill 1970). Within female respondents in this study we found no evidence of any association of lower limb

Table 11. Relationship of histological types of malignant melanoma to frequency of use of nonpermanent hair dyes

Histological type		Frequency of use of nonpermanent hair dyes			*P* value of trend
		Never	1-9 times	10+ times	
HMF:	OR	1.0	1.5	3.4	
	95% CI		0.4-5.1	1.1-10.2	0.021
SSM:	OR	1.0	0.6	0.9	
	95% CI		0.3-1.1	0.5-1.5	0.828
UCM:	OR	1.0	2.0	0.5	
	95% CI		0.8-5.0	0.2-1.5	0.233
NM:	OR	1.0	1.1	1.3	
	95% CI		0.2-6.6	0.3-5.5	0.718

Table 12. Relationship of malignant melanoma of the lower limb in women to method, age at commencement, and frequency of removal of hair from the legs (controlled for hair colour)

Risk factor	OR	95% CI	*P* value
Ever removed hair from legs	0.8	0.4-1.6	0.510
Usual method of hair removal			
Never removed hair	1.0		
Ordinary razor	0.8	0.4-1.7	0.578
Electric razor	1.4	0.4-5.0	0.629
Other methods	0.5	0.1-2.0	0.356
Ever used creams to remove hair from legs	0.6	0.3-1.4	0.211
Age at commencement of hair removal			
Never	1.0		
Ages 17+	0.5	0.2-1.1	
Ages 10-16	1.2	0.5-2.8	0.537
Frequency of hair removal			
Never	1.0		
Less than once per week	0.6	0.3-1.4	
Once per week	0.9	0.4-2.2	
More than once per week	1.2	0.4-3.4	0.614

melanoma with ever having removed hair from the legs; method of hair removal including use of creams; age at commencement of hair removal; or frequency of hair removal from the legs (see Table 12).

Tobacco

No relationship was observed between any histological type of melanoma and smoking of cigarettes, cigars or a pipe (Holman 1982). For all melanomas combined odds ratios in cigarette smokers were 0.9 (0.7-1.2) in smokers of 1-19 per day and 1.0 (0.7-1.4) in smokers of 20 or more per day (P for trend = 0.936).

Tonsillectomy, Appendectomy, and Splenectomy

The effects of past surgical excision of reticuloendothelial tissue were examined. Crude odds ratios for all melanomas were 1.0 (0.03–36.5) for splenectomy, 1.1 (0.8–1.4) for appendectomy, and 1.4 (1.1–1.8) for tonsillectomy. The association with tonsillectomy, which was strongest for SSM and UCM, was reduced slightly after control for age on arrival in Australia, owing to a higher rate of tonsillectomy in Australian children than in children from other populations who had immigrated to Australia. The adjusted odds ratios were 1.3 (1.0–1.7) for all melanomas, 1.3 (0.9–1.9) for SSM, and 1.3 (0.7–2.6) for UCM.

Other Factors

No consistent evidence of a relationship was observed between any histological type of melanoma and frequency of exposure to soaps and detergents; occupational exposure to arsenic or petroleum; use of artificial sweeteners; or consumption level of coffee or tea.

Discussion

Solar Risk Factors

There is ample evidence from this research that sunlight is a cause of malignant melanoma of the skin. The observation of increased risk in persons with poor tanning ability and other pigmentary traits typical of a low level of natural protection against the sun is consistent with previous studies (Lancaster and Nelson 1957; Gellin et al. 1969; Adam et al. 1981), and adds further to the circumstantial evidence of a causal effect of sunlight provided by this type of result.

Still more relevant, melanomas as a whole were related to the presence of actinic skin damage measured by CMT, past history of nonmelanotic skin cancer, duration of residence of migrants in Australia, and mean annual hours of bright sunlight received at the residential locations of native-born Australians. The conclusion that sunlight exposure, in the general sense, is a cause of cutaneous melanoma should now be taken as a matter of fact. Unlike the position for other skin cancers, the association between melanoma and sunlight has not been universally accepted in the past (Cutchis 1978).

While supporting a causative role of sunlight and therefore, presumably, ultraviolet radiation (UVR), our results clearly indicate that it is inappropriate to group all melanomas together in the detailed study of mechanisms whereby UVR has its effect. For this reason it is essential to consider the histological subtypes of melanoma separately.

HMF had the strongest empirical association with skin changes graded by CMT, history of nonmelanotic skin cancer, duration of residence in Australia, and mean annual sunshine hours, and was perhaps the only histological type related to the occurrence of severe sunburn. HMF was also the melanoma subtype most strongly related to poor tanning ability. These findings are consistent with HMF having a more direct relationship with sunlight exposure than the other types of melanoma. Possibly HMF and nonmelanotic skin cancers, which both occur mostly on the head and neck of middle-aged to elderly persons, share a similar causal mechanism related to cumulative dose of sunlight exposure (Holman et al. 1983).

SSM was the histological type most strongly related to the presence of benign naevi. Control subjects born in Australia or arriving before the age of 10 had more naevi on their arms than those arriving after age 10 years. We have suggested that naevus formation, and specifically the occurrence of initiated cancer cells in some naevi, at around the time of adolescence may result from exposure to UVR or other agents, and may be a critical first step in the development of SSM (Holman et al. 1983). The results relating the incidence rate of SSM to age at arrival of migrants in Australia, high residential sun exposure at ages 10–24 years, and frequency of sunbathing and type of swimsuit worn by women at ages 15–24 years, all point to a sunlight-related factor in adolescence and early adulthood. Whether the mechanism involves formation of naevi, early stimulation of naevi by UVR, or both of these, is a matter for speculation. In an examination of the interactive effects of presence of naevi and personal sun exposure habits on the rate of SSM, we found the combined effects to be generally greater than additive but less than multiplicative (Holman et al. 1985). Although the aetiological interpretation of such interaction is unclear, it has at least a public health implication in that persons with many naevi should be more careful about sun exposure habits.

The paradoxical negative relationship of SSM with total outdoor exposure, also strongest at ages 10–24 years, is consistent with other studies of melanoma and occupation (Holman et al. 1980; Beral and Robinson 1981). The intermittent exposure hypothesis (MacKie 1981; Houghton and Viola 1981; Holman et al. 1983) has been advanced to explain this paradox. The theory is supported in this study by the association of SSM with certain recreational activities involving high sun exposure; i.e., boating, fishing and sunbathing. The relationship of SSM of the trunk to clothing habits during outdoor work and swimwear in women are also supportive of the theory, especially if one accepts that exposure of the trunk is generally less frequent and better recalled than for other body sites (Holman et al. 1985). Somewhat against the intermittent exposure hypothesis was the lack of strong association of SSM with ROEP, thought a priori to be an index of occasional bursts of recreational sun exposure. If occasional bursts of sun exposure are a risk factor for SSM, stimulation of melanocytes in early adulthood rather than sunburn appears a more likely mechanism. SSM was unrelated to sunburn in these data.

Evidence associating UCM with sun exposure was much meaker than for the other histological types. Lesions categorized as UCM were those with an in situ component not recognized as having the distinct features of either HMF or SSM. Consequently, it would be reasonable to expect that this group of melanomas might be less "pure" than the more classic histoligical types with respect to certainty of diagnosis and homogeneity of causal factors.

While a role of sunlight in the causation of NM was supported by the study, the pattern of results was quite variable, partly because of the small numbers. For chronic skin reaction to sunlight, history of nonmelanotic skin cancer, and duration of residence in Australia the results for NM resembled those for HMF. However, in the case of naevi, total outdoor exposure, and ROEP, the results were more like those for SSM. We have suggested that NM represents a common end stage of the other histological types (Holman et al. 1983). If this view is correct it is reasonable that risk factors for NM should consist of a mixture of those for HMF and SSM. The apparent protective effect of sunburn on NM (and also the protective effect observed from exposure to ionizing radiation at work) is difficult to explain by any plausible physiologic mechanism and requires repetition in other studies before acceptance.

Nonsolar Risk Factors

Factors other than those related to sunlight, or sunlight protection, which received support of varying strength from our results were a family history of melanoma, ionizing radiation, oestrogenic preparations, meat consumption, alcohol, hair dyes, and tonsillectomy.

Fluorescent lighting, reproductive factors in women, polyunsaturated fats, other dietary factors, lower limb trauma through hair removal, tobacco, soaps and detergents, arsenic, petroleum, artificial sweeteners, coffee and tea received very little or no support. The results pertaining to SSM and OCP, and to serum retinol and all melanomas combined, although lacking in strenght, were not inconsistent with modest causal and protective effects, respectively. A relationship of SSM to duration of OCP use has been observed by other investigators (Holly et al. 1983). In view of this and of our borderline result associating SSM with unopposed oestrogenic preparations, we are reluctant to dismiss the SSM-OCP relationship out of hand. Similarly, a protective effect of high serum retinol on the rates of several types of cancer has been described (Peto et al. 1981), and has hence received considerable prior credibility.

A positive family history in a blood relative was a definite risk factor which, for the most part, was independent of number of nevi and pigmentary traits. The absence of increased risk in persons with an affected relative by marriage argues against an explanation on the grounds of shared environment. It appears, therefore, that specific genetic factors may exist which predispose to the development of melanoma.

Nonpermanent hair dyes and occupational exposure to ionizing radiation appeared to increase the incidence rate of HMF. Given that some nonpermanent hair dyes have contained aromatic colouring agents which are carcinogenic in experimental animals, and the carcinogenic properties of X-rays are well known, we have little difficulty in accepting that the relationships between HMF and these agents have biological plausibility. We are mindful, however, that the result pertaining to exposure to ionizing radiation at work was of borderline significance and was inconsistent with results obtained from recording of therapeutic expsure to X-rays.

The findings of associations of UCM with high alcohol intake and NM with meat consumption, and the effects of tonsillectomy on the rates of SSM and UCM are mainly new results, which warrant further investigation in future studies. A relationship of melanomas as a whole to intake of spirits was observed in data from the Third U.S. National Cancer Survey (Williams and Horm 1977). With the comparative sparsity of causal factors for UCM identified elsewhere, the possibility exists that a proportion of UCM may be an alcohol-related variant of melanoma. However, this result and those relating to meat consumption and tonsillectomy were borderline in strength and consistency, and therefore we do not wish to overempasize their importance.

Benign Naevi

The strong relationship between non-HMF melanoma and naevi counted on the subjects' arms, as well as the evidence that a greater number of naevi may be induced in persons resident in a sunny climate during their youth, has already been discussed. Whether on this basis naevi should be regarded as a solar-related risk factor is a moot point. The proper perspective is probably to regard them as percursor lesions, which may arise via several mechanisms, including genetically determined mechanisms as in the dysplastic naevus syndrome, familial type (Greene et al. 1980).

It is our view that further advances in our understanding of melanoma causation would be well served by intensified study of the epidemiology, natural history, and constitutional and environmental determinants of benign naevi. To this end a cohort study of the development of naevi in children and a detailed investigation of dysplastic naevi in relation to family history are under way in Western Australia at present.

Acknowledgements. The authors are grateful to the people of Western Australia and to the many medical practitioners, nurses and other colleagues who made this research possible.

References

Adam SA, Sheaves JK, Wright NH, et al (1981) A case-control study of the possible association between oral contraceptives and malignant melanoma. Br J Cancer 44: 45–50
Armstrong BK (1985) Epidemiology of cancer in Australia. Med J Aust 142: 124–130
Beagley J, Gibson IM (1980) Changes in skin condition in relation to degree of exposure to ultraviolet light. School of Biology, Western Australian Institute of Technology, Perth
Beral V, Robinson N (1981) The relationship of malignant melanoma, basal and squamous skin cancers to indoor and outdoor work. Br J Cancer 44: 886–891
Beral V, Evans S, Shaw H, Milton G (1982) Malignant melanoma and exposure to fluorescent lights. Lancet 2: 290–293
Breslow NE, Day NE (1980) Statistical methods in cancer research, vol 1. The analysis of case-control studies. IARC Sci Publ 32
Cutchis P (1978) On the linkage of solar ultraviolet radiation to skin cancer. Institute of Defence Analyses Paper P-1342, U.S. Department of Transportation, Washington DC
English DR, Rouse IL, Zhong X, et al. (1985) Cutaneous malignant melanoma and fluorescent lighting. JNCI 74: 1191–1197
Gellin GA, Kopf AW, Garfinkel L (1969) Malignant melanoma. A controlled study of possibly associated factors. Arch Dermatol 99: 43–48
Greene MH, Clark WH Jr, Tucker MA, et al. (1980) Precursor naevi in cutaneous malignant melanoma. A proposed nomenclature. Lancet 2: 1024
Hoar SK, Morrison AS, Cole P, Silverman DT (1980) An occupation and exposure linkage system for the study of occupational carcinogensis. J Occup Med 22: 722–726
Holly EA, Weiss NS, Liff JM (1983) Cutaneous melanoma in relation to exogenous hormones and reproductive factors. JNCI 70: 827–883
Holman CDJ (1982) Risk factors in the causation of human malignant melanoma of the skin. PhD thesis, University of Western Australia, Perth. University Microfilms International, Ann Arbor, Mich
Holman CDJ, Armstrong BK (1982) Distribution of malignant melanoma on the body surface. Br J Cancer 45: 317
Holman CDJ, Armstrong BK (1983) Hutchinson's melanotic freckle melanoma associated with non-permanent hair dyes. Br J Cancer 48: 599–601
Holman CDJ, Armstrong BK (1984a) Pigmentary traits, ethnic origin, benign nevi, and family history as risk factors for cutaneous malignant melanoma. JNCI 72: 257–266
Holman CDJ, Armstrong BK (1984b) Cutaneous malignant melanoma and indicators of total accumulated exposure to the sun: An analysis separating histogenetic types. JNCI 73: 75–82
Holman CDJ, Mulroney CD, Armstrong BK (1980) Epidemiology of preinvasive and invasive malignant melanoma in Western Australia. Int J Cancer 25: 317–323
Holman CDJ, Armstrong BK, Heenan PJ (1983) Guest editorial: A theory of the etiology and pathogenesis of human cutaneous malignant melanoma. JNCI 71: 651–656
Holman CDJ, Armstrong BK, Evans PR, et al. (1984a) Relationship of solar keratosis and history of skin cancer to objective measures of actinic skin damage. Br J Dermatol 110: 129–138

Holman CDJ, Armstrong BK, Heenan PJ (1984b) Cutaneous malignant melanoma in women: Exogeneous sex hormones and reproduktive factors. Br J Cancer 50: 673-680

Holman CDJ, Armstrong BK, Heenan PJ (1985) Relationship of cutaneous malignant melanoma to individual sunlight exposure habits. JNCI (in press)

Houghton AN, Viola MV (1981) Solar radiation and malignant melanoma of the skin. J Am Acad Dermatol 5: 477-483

Lancaster HO, Nelson J (1957) Sunlight as a cause of melanoma: A clinical survey. Med J Aust 1: 452-456

Landsberg H (1966) World maps of climatology. Total hours of sunshine (annual). Springer, Berlin Heidelberg New York

Lee JAH, Merrill JM (1970) Sunlight and the aetiology of malignant melanoma: A synthesis. Med J Aust 2: 846-851

MacKie RM (1981) The role of sunlight in the aetiology of cutaneous malignant melanoma Clin Exp Dermatol 6: 407-410

Mackie BS, Johnson AR, Mackie LE, Fogerty AC, Ferris M, Baxter RI (1980) Dietary polyunsaturated fats and malignant melanoma. Med J Aust 1: 159-162

McGovern VJ, Mihm MC Jr, Bailly C, et al. (1973) The classification of malignant melanoma and its histologic reporting. Cancer 32: 1446-1457

Peto R, Doll R, Buckley JD, Sporn MB (1981) Can dietary beta-carotene materially reduce human cancer rates? Nature 290: 201-208

Thomas DC (1980) Program "RISK". Department of Epidemiology and Health, McGill University, Montreal

Williams RR, Horm JW (1977) Association of cancer sites with tobacco and alcohol consumption and socioeconomic status of patients: interview study from the Third national Cancer Survey. JNCI 58: 525-547

*Risk Factors for Cutaneous Malignant Melanoma: The Western Canada Melanoma Study**

R. P. Gallagher, J. M. Elwood, and G. B. Hill

Cancer Control Agency of British Columbia, 600 West 10th Avenue, Vancouver, B.C. V5Z 4E6, Canada

Introduction

Over the past 3 decades the incidence and mortality from melanoma in Canada, the United Kingdom, United States, Australia and the Nordic countries has increased dramatically (Elwood and Lee 1974; Kopf et al. 1984; Little et al. 1980; Magnus 1977; Muir and Nectoux 1982). A number of factors have been linked aetiologically with melanoma, including host factors such as light skin, hair and eye colour (Elwood et al. 1984; Gellin et al. 1969; Holman and Armstrong 1984a; Lancaster and Nelson 1957). There is evidence that risk of melanoma is related to sunlight exposure (Elwood and Hislop 1982; Holman et al. 1983), although the relationship is obviously not a simple one. It has been suggested that intermittent heavy sunlight exposure may be more important than constant dose in risk of superficial spreading melanomas, and this theory is supported by findings of similarity of incidence rates by unit area on usually and intermittently exposed body sites (Elwood and Gallagher 1983).

In addition to host pigmentation factors and sunlight exposure, there is some evidence that use of oral contraceptives may place women at a higher risk of melanoma (Beral et al. 1977, 1984; Holly et al. 1983).

This report summarizes findings to date from the Western Canada Melanoma Study, based on 595 study subjects aged 20-79 with superficial spreading, nodular or unclassified melanomas and their matched controls. Data on lentigo maligna cases will be analysed separately in future reports.

Methods

Reports of all newly diagnosed, histologically confirmed cases of malignant melanoma seen in Western Canada (British Columbia, Alberta, Saskatchewan, Manitoba) from 1 April 1979 to 31 March 1981 were obtained through the cancer registries of each province. All available patients aged 20-79 were approached for interview. Each patient was matched by age (±2 years) and sex with a control subject selected at random from medical insurance plan lists of subscribers. The medical insurance plans cover virtually the en-

* Financial support for this study was provided by Health & Welfare Canada (NHRDP 6610-1203-53), the National Cancer Institute of Canada, and the Alberta Heritage Trust Fund

Recent Results in Cancer Research. Vol 102

tire adult population of each province. Patients and controls were interviewed in their homes by trained interviewers using a standardized questionnaire. Information was obtained on a number of variables, including host pigmentation and reaction to sunlight, residence, occupational history, recreational activities with specific reference to sunlight exposure, medical history, chronic drug use, family history, diet, smoking and alcohol consumption; and for women, reproductive history and use of oral contraceptives and menopausal oestrogens.

Skin and hair colour were determined by direct comparison with prosthesis and wigmakers samples, made up specifically for the project. Skin colour was assessed twice on each of a sun-exposed area (dorsum of each hand) and a non-sun-exposed area (upper inner aspect of each arm). Eye colour was recorded on the questionnaire form by the interviewer from direct observation.

In the event that hair colour had greyed with age, subjects were asked to indicate from the samples their natural hair colour in childhood and as a young adult. Information on sensitivity to sunlight and tanning and sunburning both as an adult and as a child were collected. In addition, subjects were queried about degree of skin freckling in childhood.

A standardized abstract of the medical record was made for each patient and included data on symptoms, treatment and recurrences. Pathological slides were reviewed in a standardized manner by one of two reference pathologists (Dr. A. J. Worth, Dr. W. S. Wood) at the Cancer Control Agency of British Columbia. Pathological slides were unavailable for 20% of the patients, and in these cases the original pathology report was used.

In the 2-year period of case intake, 904 patients with primary cutaneous melanomatous lesions were registered, 801 of whom were age eligible (20–79) for the study. Of these, 665 (83%) were interviewed along with matched controls. Of those cases not interviewed, 21 were dead and 40 could not be located. In a further 21 cases the subjects' physician felt that an interview would not be in the patients' best interests, and the remaining 54 cases declined participation in the study. Of the 665 cases interviewed, 56 had lentigo maligna and 14 acral lentiginous melanoma. Since the clinical and epidemiological features of these subtypes may be quite different from those of other melanomas (Clark and Mihm 1969; Holman et al. 1983; Holman and Armstrong 1984b; McGovern et al. 1979), the analyses in this paper are restricted to the remaining 595 cases. Of these, 415 had superficial spreading melanoma, 128 nodular melanoma, 23 unclassified melanoma and 29 borderline melanomas. Of the 595 cases 234 were male and 361 female.

In Manitoba, Saskatchewan and Alberta, the study co-ordinators were allowed direct access to provincial microfiche listings of medical plan subscribers, and subjects selected as potential controls were telephoned. Of those contacted, 59% agreed to co-operate. In British Columbia, a letter requesting participation was sent out by the Medical Services Commission, and subjects were required to return a completed consent form before contact by study personnel was allowed. No telephone contact was permitted. This gave a response rate of 48%. The low response rate for each province was attributed largely to the fact that selected individuals could not be contacted at the addresses given by the provincial medical plans. Potential controls who declined to participate did so largely because of the length of the required interview (1.5–2.0 h).

The analysis of data was conducted in a similar fashion for each of the topic areas examined. Crude associations were computed, based on matched pairs, with odds ratios as an estimate of relative risk. Then, to adjust for the effect of other variables on significant associations detected, a multiple logistic model based on matched pairs was fitted according to the procedures of Breslow and Day (1980). Statistically significant results were those where the two-sided P-value was less than 0.05 based on the change in log likelihood for the multivariate model. In some analyses, such as those involving sunburn and suntan histories, crude relative risks were adjusted for possible confounding by the Mantel - Haenszel method (Mantel and Haenszel 1959) to minimise the loss of subjects with missing suntan or sunburn information.

Results

Host Pigmentation

Differences were seen between cases and controls for hair colour, colour of skin on the non-sun-exposed areas of the upper arm, and eye colour (Table 1). In general, melanoma patients had lighter colouring than controls. Against subjects with black hair, those with blonde hair had a crude relative risk of 9.7. The corresponding relative risk was 3.4 for subjects with light compared with dark skin, and 1.6 for blue- compared with brown-eyed patients. Each of these factors considered alone was statistically significant. After adjustment of each factor for the effect of other pigmentation variables (freckling, sun reaction, frequency of childhood sunburn, and ethnic origin), blonde hair was associated with a relative risk of 7.1 compared with dark hair, and light skin colour had a relative risk of 2.4

Table 1. Pigmentation factors, ethnic origin and risk of melanoma in 595 subjects and matched controls

Factor	Category	% Cases	RR Crude[a]	RR Adjusted[b]
Hair colour	Black	3	1.0	1.0
	Dark brown	39	2.6	2.5
	Brown	41	3.4	2.8
	Red and light brown	13	5.0	3.7
	Blonde	5	9.7	7.1
				$x^2=20.3$, $P<0.001$
Skin colour	Dark	2	1.0	1.0
	Mid	28	2.2	1.9
	Light	70	3.4	2.4
				$x^2=6.8$, $P<0.05$
Eye colour	Brown	19	1.0	1.0
	Green, grey, hazel	27	1.4	1.1
	Blue	54	1.6	1.2
				$x^2=4.3$, $P=$NS
Ethnic origin	English	40	1.0	1.0
	Celtic, Scandinavian	19	0.9	0.7
	Western European	24	0.7	0.7
	Eastern and Southern European	5	0.5	0.6
	Other	21	0.9	1.1
				$x^2=9.5$, $P<0.05$

[a] Crude relative risks based on matched pairs and *P* values
[b] Relative risks for each factor adjusted for other pigmentation factors and for freckling, childhood sunburn and ethnic origin by matched logistic analysis

Table 2. Childhood freckling and sunburn, and risk of melanoma in 595 cases and matched controls

Factor	Category	% Cases	RR Crude[a]	RR Adjusted[b]
Freckles in childhood	None	45	1.0	1.0
	Few	13	1.3	1.3
	Some	21	1.6	1.4
	Many	21	2.6	2.1
				$x^2=25.1$, $P<0.001$
Childhood sunburn	Rare or mild	24	1.0	1.0
	Moderate or infrequent	27	1.4	1.1
	Severe or frequent	49	1.9	1.3
				$x^2=1.8$, $P=$ NS

[a] Crude relative risks based on matched pairs and *P* values
[b] Relative risks for each factor adjusted for other pigmentation factors and for freckling, childhood sunburn and ethnic origin by matched logistic analysis

compared with dark skin. After adjustment for other host variables, the relative risk for blue eyes as against brown eyes fell to 1.2, which was no longer statistically significant. Analyses by sex showed no significant differences.

Ethnic origin proved to be an independent predictor of risk, with southern Europeans having a much lower risk of melanoma than those of English origin. The analyses for pigmentation factors were repeated including data on occupational, recreational and vacation sunlight exposure in the model. The risk estimates for pigmentation factors were not substantially altered by these adjustments.

Freckling and Sunburn in Childhood

Subjects who reported a great many freckles in childhood had a significantly elevated crude risk of melanoma (RR=2.6) compared with those who had no freckling. The risk dropped slightly but was still statistically significant even after adjustment for other host and pigmentation factors (RR=2.1) (Table 2).

Respondents were asked about their history of frequency of sunburns in childhood, and on univariate analysis those with frequent or severe sunburns showed a significantly elevated risk (RR=1.9) in comparison with those having rare or mild sunburns. However, when pigmentation factors and skin sun reaction were taken into account, the relative risk dropped (RR=1.3) and became statistically nonsignificant. Inclusion of ultraviolet light exposure (sunlight) in the model did not materially alter relative risks.

Skin Reaction to Sun

Respondents were asked how their skin reacted to strong sunlight in the first few days of summer exposure. Compared with subjects who would "usually get a brown suntan without burning", those who "only got a sunburn and rarely a tan" had an elevated risk of melanoma (RR=2.3) (Table 3). After adjustment for host pigmentation characteristics, the relative risk fell somewhat (RR=1.7), but was still significantly elevated.

Table 3. Skin reaction to sun and risk of melanoma in 595 cases and matched controls

Factor	Category	% Cases	RR Crude[a]	RR Adjusted[b]
Skin reaction to sunlight	Tan, no burn	31	1.0	1.0
	Tan with protection	13	2.0	1.8
	Burn then tan	42	1.9	1.5
	Burn only	14	2.3	1.7
				$x^2 = 12.4$, $P < 0.01$

[a] Crude relative risks based on matched pairs and *P* values

[b] Relative risks adjusted for hair colour, skin colour, freckling and ethnic origin by matched logistic analysis

Sunburn, Suntan and Skin Reaction to Sun

Since skin reaction to sunlight was a predictor of melanoma risk independent of host pigmentation, we elected to analyse data on suntan and sunburn to try to separate the *propensity* of skin to tan or burn as determined by the skin reaction; as opposed to the *actual* burning and tanning history of subjects.

History of sunburn was recorded from detailed recreation and vacation histories. Study subjects were asked about vacations of one week or more in which they were out in the sun for considerably more time than usual or were exposed to stronger sunlight than usual. Subjects were asked about whether they developed a sunburn during these times. The severity of the sunburn was graded 1-3 in severity as “rare, very mild, or never”, “moderate or infrequent” or “severe or frequent burn”. The responses were recorded for each of four body areas: hands and face, upper limbs, lower limbs and trunk. Severity scores were weighted by body areas burned and a sunburn index was created for each patient (Elwood et al. 1985b).

Subjects were questioned about their usual degree of suntan in the context of recreational activities in winter and summer, for the four body areas by decade of life. Suntan was graded from 1 to 3 as “rarely any suntan,” “mild or occasional tan” or “usually had a deep tan”.

On crude analysis, risk of melanoma was found to be associated with degree of past sunburn, a “very severe” history of sunburn conferring a relative risk of 1.8 (Table 4). However, when the relationship was controlled for the effect of skin reaction to sun the relationship between sunburn and melanoma was no longer significant. Reversal of the analysis with control of the association between melanoma and skin reaction to sun for the effect of sunburn history produced no difference in the previously detected independent association between melanoma and skin reaction. Thus the propensity of the skin to sunburn appears to be more important than actual sunburn history in the development of elevated risk of melanoma.

Examination of the suntan data revealed an inverse association on univariate analysis between risk of melanoma and degree of suntan (Table 5). Subjects with a mild tan or no tan summer or winter had a significantly elevated risk of melanoma (RR = 2.0). When the association was re-examined controlling for skin reaction to sunlight the inverse relationship between melanoma and degree of suntan became nonsignificant. Thus, degree of suntan also appears to be less important in malignant melanoma than the skin sensitivity; that is, the ability of the skin to tan rather than burn in the sun.

Table 4. History of sunburn and risk of melanoma in 479 cases and 445 controls[a]

Factor	Category	% Cases	RR Crude[b]	RR Adjusted[c]
Vacation sunburn score	≤4 Mild	52	1.0	1.0
	5-7 Moderate	20	1.2	1.0
	8-9 Severe	17	1.3	1.1
	10-12 Very severe	11	1.8	1.4
			x^2(trend) = 6.4, $P<0.02$	x^2(trend) = 1.3, $P>0.2$

[a] Results are based on 479 cases and 445 controls, since 116 patients and 150 controls were excluded due to missing data
[b] Crude relative risks based on matched pairs and p values
[c] Relative risks adjusted for skin reaction to sunlight by Mantel-Haenszel method

Table 5. Suntan and risk of melanoma in 569 cases and 533 controls[a]

Factor	Category[b]	% Cases	RR Crude[c]	RR Adjusted[d]
Usual degree of suntan	1 Moderate/deep	6	1.0	1.0
	2 Mild/deep	32	1.5	1.4
	3 Mild/moderate	37	1.7	1.4
	4 Mild/mild	25	2.0	1.6
			x^2(trend) = 8.4, $P<0.01$	x^2(trend) = 3.0, $P>0.1$

[a] Results are based on 569 cases and 553 controls, since 26 patients and 38 controls were excluded due to missing data
[b] Suntan categories are: 1, moderate winter tan/deep summer tan; 2 mild winter tan/deep summer tan; 3 mild winter tan/moderate summer tan; 4 mild winter tan/mild summer tan
[c] Crude relative risks based on matched pairs and *P* values
[d] Relative risks adjusted for skin reaction to sunlight by Mantel - Haenszel method

Sunlight (Ultraviolet Light) Exposure

Prior research has indicated a relationship between risk of melanoma and exposure to sunlight, but the character of the relationship is still in question. Our study hypothesis was that melanoma risk increases with heavy intermittent sunlight exposure to skin which is normally little exposed to the sun; while chronic sun exposure at a constant dose has relatively little effect. We measured sunlight in occupational, recreational and vacation contexts, as described in a previous detailed report (Elwood et al. 1985 a).

Occupational sun exposure has been taken to be indicative of chronic constant exposure, while vacation and recreation exposures, particularly summer exposures, were analysed as surrogates for intermittent sunshine exposure. We evaluated risk of melanoma by each type of sunlight exposure.

Occupational Sunlight Exposure. Compared with subjects having no occupational exposure, those with mild exposure of 1-99 whole-body equivalent hours (EH) per year (corresponding to about 8 h per week of exposure) had a significantly increased risk of melanoma (RR = 1.8) after adjustment for host factors (Table 6). However, at higher exposures no increase was seen, the risk being similar to that of the lowest exposure group. The signifi-

Table 6. Occupational sunlight exposure and risk of melanoma in 595 cases and matched controls

Factor	Equivalent hours of exposure[a]	Approx. hours per week[a]	% Cases	RR Adjusted[b]
Occupational sunlight exposure	<1	0	24	1.0
	1-99	1-8	33	1.8
	100-199	9-16	17	1.0
	200-399	17-32	15	0.9
	400+	33+	12	0.9
				$\chi^2 = 16.4$, $P < 0.01$

[a] One whole-body equivalent hour (EH) of exposure represents 1 h of sun exposure to the whole body surface. Recorded exposures were converted to EH using estimates of proportion of body area exposed. "Approx. hours" means the number of hours per week of actual exposure with typical clothing for the given EH to be achieved

[b] Relative risks adjusted for hair colour, skin colour, freckling, and ethnic origin by matched logistic analysis

Table 7. Recreational sunlight exposure and risk of melanoma in 595 cases and matched controls

Factor	Equivalent hours of exposure[a]	Approx. hours per week[a]	% Cases	RR Adjusted[b]
Recreational Sunlight Exposure Beach type activities (Summer season)	<1	0	29	1.0
	1-19	<1	15	1.1
	20-79	1-4	28	1.7
	80-159	5-8	15	1.8
	160+	9+	13	1.7
				$\chi^2 = 15.3$, $P < 0.01$

[a] One whole body equivalent hour (EH) of exposure represents 1 h of sun exposure to the whole body surface. Recorded exposures were converted to EH using estimates of proportion of body area exposed. "Approx. hours" means the number of hours per week of actual exposure with typical clothing for the given EH to be achieved

[b] Relative risks adjusted for hair colour, skin colour, freckling and ethnic origin by matched logistic analysis

cant chi-square value was caused by the elevated melanoma risk (RR = 1.8) for those with an EH value of 1-99. Otherwise, no rising trend was seen for higher levels of occupational sun exposure.

Recreational Sunlight Exposure. Recreational sunlight exposure was assessed in terms of participation in outdoor activities. For summer beach-type activities (swimming, water activities, sunbathing) the risk of melanoma was increased in subjects with greater than 20 EH, equivalent to approximately 1-4 h sunlight exposure per week over the summer months (Table 7). The elevated risk persisted after adjustment for host factors, although its value declined slightly (RR = 1.7). Examination of other summer activities in which light clothing was worn (baseball, soccer, tennis) demonstrated a similar, but less marked trend to that seen in beach activities. No statistically significant association was seen with any group of winter activities.

Table 8. Vacation sunlight exposure and risk of melanoma in 595 cases and matched controls

Factor	Equivalent hours of exposure[a]	Approx. hours per week[a]	% Cases	RR Adjusted[b]
Vacation	<1	0	33	1.0
Sunlight	1–6	<1	25	0.9
Exposure	7–19	1–4	13	0.9
Beach type	20–39	5–8	15	1.9
activities	40+	9+	14	1.5
(Summer season)				$\chi^2=15.4$, $P<0.01$

[a] One whole-body equivalent hour (EH) of exposure represents 1 h of sun exposure to the whole body surface. Recorded exposures were converted to EH using estimates of proportion of body area exposed. "Approx. hours" means the number of hours per week of actual exposure with typical clothing for the given EH to be achieved

[b] Relative risks adjusted for hair colour, skin colour, freckling, and ethnic origin by matched logistic analysis

Vacation Sunlight Exposure. Sun exposure during vacations was also assessed for different activity groups and for summer and winter vacations separately. Risk of melanoma increased with exposure to beach type activities in summer vacations, to reach a relative risk of 1.9 with 20–39 EH, equivalent to 4–8 h per day of exposure during a 1-week vacation (Table 8). Although only 30 cases and 16 controls had substantial exposure to vacation sun through ice and snow activities during winter vacations, the relative risk associated with these activities was significantly elevated (RR=2.0, $P=0.05$).

Total Sunlight Exposure

Information on each of the sources of sunlight was combined into a single category to assess the relationship between cumulative sunlight exposure and risk of melanoma, but no trend was seen and overall there was no statistically significant association between total sunlight exposure and risk of melanoma.

Oral Contraceptive Use in Females

A number of studies have examined the relationship between use of exogenous oestrogens and risk of melanoma. Several studies have found an association between melanoma and use of oral contraceptives (Beral et al. 1977, 1984); however, a number of other studies have demonstrated marginal associations or no association (Adam et al. 1981; Bain et al. 1982; Helmrich et al. 1984; Holman et al. 1984). Holly et al. (1983) also demonstrated an elevated risk of superficial spreading melanoma in women with late age at first birth (⩾31 years). The Western Canada Melanoma Study examined both reproductive factors and use of exogenous oestrogens.

Data on a total of 361 female cases and their matched controls were available for analysis. Of these cases, 269 were superficial spreading, 66 were nodular and 26 were unclassified melanomas.

Our analysis for oral contraceptives was restricted to women aged 20–69 at diagnosis. Older women were excluded as they would have reached menopausal age prior to the in-

Table 9. Oral contraceptive use and risk of melanoma in 333 cases and controls aged 20–69 years

		Not used	<1 year	1-4 years	5+ years	*P* value
All melanomas (333 cases)	% Cases	42	10	23	23	$\chi^2=1.6$, NS
	RR adjusted[a]	1.0	1.0	0.9	0.8	
Superficial spreading melanoma (250 cases)	% Cases	44	10	21	25	$\chi^2=0.5$, NS
	RR adjusted[a]	1.0	1.1	1.1	0.9	
Nodular melanoma (59 cases)	% Cases	42	15	32	12	$\chi^2=2.2$, NS
	RR adjusted[a]	1.0	1.5	1.0	0.3	

[a] Each RR adjusted for skin colour, hair colour, freckling and educational status by matched logistic analysis

troduction of oral contraceptives to the market. No association was seen between use of oral contraceptives and risk of melanoma for all melanomas combined or superficial spreading or nodular lesions analysed separately (Table 9). Further analyses controlling for numbers of live births also showed no association. A series of separate analyses were performed for women aged 20–39 and 40–69, and no relationship was demonstrated. No association was found with years since "last use of oral contraceptives", even in women who had ceased using the preparations 10 or more years prior to diagnosis.

Other exogenous oestrogen use (mainly menopausal oestrogens) was not associated with either elevated or reduced risk of subsequent melanoma (Gallagher et al. 1985).

Sunlamp Usage

Subjects were questioned about the frequency and duration of sunlamp use, as well as the body sites it was used on. No association was found between sunlamp use and subsequent risk of melanoma ($\chi^2=6.1$, 5 d.f., P= NS). Separate analysis by sex showed no relationship for either males and females. A further set of analyses separating body sites on which the sunlamp was used (face and neck, trunk, arms, legs) also showed no association with risk of melanoma.

Prior Skin Problems

Subjects were asked about a variety of skin conditions possibly related to subsequent development of cutaneous melanoma (Table 10).

Acne. No association was seen between presence of acne and subsequent risk of melanoma. When separate analyses were conducted by sex, data on females showed no association, however, a relative risk of 1.5 was seen on males who had had prior acne, although the risk was not statistically significant ($\chi^2=3.1$, 1 d.f., $P=0.08$). Examination of data on age of development of the condition and its severity or treatment produced no significant findings.

Psoriasis. Prior psoriasis was examined in study subjects as a possible risk factor for melanoma. No association was seen for both sexes combined ($\chi^2=1.2$, 1 d.f., P= NS) or for either sex separately.

Table 10. Prior skin problems and risk of melanoma in 595 cases and controls

Factor	Category	% Cases	% Controls	Crude RR[a]
Acne	No	76	76	1.0
	Yes	24	24	1.0
				$\chi^2 = 0.01$, $P=$ NS
Psoriasis	No	93	95	1.0
	Yes	7	5	1.4
				$\chi^2 = 1.2$, $P=$ NS
Dermatitis	No	72	28	1.0
	Yes	68	32	0.8
				$\chi^2 = 2.5$, $P=$ NS

[a] Relative risks based on matched pairs and *P* values

Dermatitis. No association was seen between risk of melanoma and prior self-reported dermatitis ($\chi^2 = 2.5$, 1 *d.f.*, $P=$ NS). Subjects were asked whether specific materials caused the rash or dermatitis, but no particular agents were found to be important. Analysis by sex showed no association with melanoma.

Vitiligo and Xeroderma pigmentosum. Only one subject in the study had been diagnosed as having xeroderma pigmentosum. This subject was a woman with melanoma, who had had multiple prior basal cell carcinomas and several melanomas. She died of her melanoma before our study ended.

Subjects were also asked whether they "had ever been told by a physician that they had vitiligo". Only five patients and four controls answered in the affirmative, and no association was seen with subsequent risk of melanoma. No attempt was made to verify the diagnosis of vertiligo.

Viral Diseases

Subjects were questioned about previous viral diseases, including mumps, infectious mononucleosis, chickenpox, rubeola, and rubella (Table 11). No association was seen with any of the diseases, with the exception of rubella, which was slightly more common in patients than controls. Analyses by sex showed the association was confined to female patients (RR = 1.5, $\chi^2 = 4.9$, 1 *d.f.*, $P = 0.03$). No corresponding increased risk was seen in males and it seems likely that the finding may be a chance occurrence due to multiple testing.

Other Chronic Diseases and Surgery

Prior chronic diseases, including diabetes, hypertension, peptic ulcer, arthritis, diseases of the gallbladder, and neurofibromatosis were examined in cases and controls (Table 12).

Table 11. Prior viral diseases and risk of melanoma in 595 cases and controls

Factor	Category	% Cases	% Controls	Crude RR[a]
Mumps	No	26	27	1.0
	Yes	74	73	1.1
				$\chi^2=0.4$, $P=$ NS
Infectious mononucleosis	No	93	95	1.0
	Yes	7	5	1.5
				$\chi^2=1.9$, $P=$ NS
Chickenpox	No	17	21	1.0
	Yes	83	80	1.2
				$\chi^2=1.3$, $P=$ NS
Rubeola	No	21	22	1.0
	Yes	78	78	1.0
				$\chi^2=0.05$, $P=$ NS
Rubella	No	31	39	1.0
	Yes	68	61	1.4
				$\chi^2=6.2$, $P=0.01$

[a] Relative risks based on matched pairs and *P*-values

Table 12. Prior chronic diseases and risk of melanoma in 595 cases and controls

Factor	Category	% Cases	% Controls	Crude RR[a]
Diabetes	No	96	95	1.0
	Yes	4	5	0.8
				$\chi^2=0.2$, $P=$ NS
Hypertension	No	84	81	1.0
	Yes	16	19	0.8
				$\chi^2=1.2$, $P=$ NS
Gallbladder disease	No	85	86	1.0
	Yes	15	14	1.1
				$\chi^2=0.2$, $P=$ NS
Peptic ulcer	No	93	90	1.0
	Yes	7	10	0.7
				$\chi^2=2.3$, $P=$ NS
Arthritis (any type)	No	87	83	1.0
	Yes	13	17	0.7
				$\chi^2=3.0$, $P=$ NS

[a] Relative risks based on matched pairs and *P* values

No significant associations were seen with risk of malignant melanoma. Subjects were also questioned about previous tonsillectomy and appendectomy, but no significant associations were seen with risk of malignant melanoma.

Smoking

Since tobacco is a common carcinogen, the study examined the consumption of plain and filter cigarettes and of pipe tobacco and cigars. No association was seen with any form of smoking (cigarettes: $\chi^2=0.15$, 1 *d.f.*, $P=$ NS). Males and females were analysed separately and a further analysis by pack years was conducted for cases and controls within 10-year age groups, but no significant findings emerged.

Table 13. Frequency of consumption of different foods and risk of melanoma in 595 cases and controls

Food	High[a] ←	Consumption[b] RR			Low[a] →	Significance level
Vegetables (uncooked)	1.0	1.0	0.9	0.6	0.9	χ^2 (trend) = 1.2 $P=$ NS
Vegetables (cooked)	1.0	1.0	1.2	1.0	0.8	χ^2 (trend) = 0.1 $P=$ NS
Beef	1.0	1.1	1.2	0.6	1.5	χ^2 (trend) = 0.4 $P=$ NS
Other meat	1.0	1.2	1.3	0.8	1.0	χ^2 (trend) = 0.01 $P=$ NS
Smoked or barbecued foods	1.0	1.0	1.0	1.0	1.0	χ^2 (trend) = 0.01 $P=$ NS
Fish	1.0	0.4	0.6	0.4	0.6	χ^2 (trend) = 2.1 $P=$ NS
Eggs	1.0	1.5	1.5	1.1	0.8	χ^2 (trend) = 0.2 $P=$ NS
Milk	1.0	1.1	1.1	0.8	1.0	χ^2 (trend) = 0.1 $P=$ NS
Cheese	1.0	0.9	0.8	0.9	0.7	χ^2 (trend) = 2.2 $P=$ NS
Butter	1.0	1.3	0.6	1.1	0.9	χ^2 (trend) = 1.1 $P=$ NS
Margarine	1.0	1.2	2.8	0.6	1.1	χ^2 (trend) = 1.0 $P=$ NS

[a] Index based on frequency of consumption from high (at least once per day) to low (less than once per month or never)
[b] Measured as current consumption on a food frequency questionnaire

Alcohol Consumption

No significant differences were seen between cases and controls for consumption of wine, beer or spirits. A composite of all alcohol consumption was also not associated with increased risk of melanoma. Analysis by sex and by age group showed no association.

Diet

Diet is thought to be related to the incidence of a number of common cancers in Western countries, and so we recorded data on consumption of a number of foodstuffs among melanoma patients and controls. Subjects were queried about levels of consumption of fresh, canned and cooked vegetables, beef, other red meats, fish, smoked or barbecued foods, butter, milk, cheese and margarine. Most dietary items were chosen because they have been associated singly or in food groups as putative risk or protective factors for other tumours. No significant differences were seen for any food (Table 13).

Consumption of coffee, tea and use of artificial sweeteners was examined for all subjects, but no association was seen with any of these foods.

Subjects were queried about whether their diet had changed in the 10 years prior to interview. Only 15 cases and 22 controls reported any major change in their diet. Thus, dietary intake appears to have been fairly consistent, and recent dietary changes do not appear to have confounded our analysis.

Discussion

Of the variables examined in the Western Canada Melanoma Study, the most important concerned host pigmentation and ethnic origin, skin reaction to sunlight, and the effect of intermittent versus constant sunlight exposure.

Of the pigmentation variables, hair colour demonstrated the strongest relationship with risk of melanoma. Light colouring of non-sun-exposed skin conferred additional risk. Light eye colour, although related to risk of melanoma on crude analysis, was found to be a statistically nonsignificant factor when the analysis was controlled for other pigmentation variables. The findings of increased risk of melanoma in fair-haired and fair-skinned individuals accords with descriptive data (Waterhouse et al. 1982) and results of a number of analytic studies (Gellin et al. 1969; Holman and Armstrong 1984a).

Our study additionally found an association between ethnic origin and risk of melanoma, which was independent of host pigmentation characteristics. Subjects of eastern and southern European extraction (defined as Hungary, Czechoslovakia, Poland and Italy) have a lower risk than individuals of English, Celtic or Scandinavian descent. The finding of lower risk for southern and eastern Europeans is in agreement with relatively low melanoma incidence rates in these areas (Waterhouse et al. 1982).

The association with number of freckles seen in the Western Canada Study might have been expected, given the known association of freckling with light skin colour (Nicholls 1968), but it appears that freckling is an independent risk factor even after adjustment for other host factors. In a Norwegian study, Klepp and Magnus (1979) reported that their patients developed freckles more easily than controls. In addition, several recent studies have identified the presence of numerous benign naevi as a strong risk factor for cutaneous melanoma (Beral et al. 1983; Holman and Armstrong 1984a; Swerdlow et al. 1984).

The direct relationship between melanoma and freckling suggests that freckles and naevi have an important role in the pathogenesis of melanoma. Results from our own study, and those of Holman and others are consistent with the hypothesis that superficial spreading and nodular melanomas develop from naevi (McGovern et al. 1967) and that the two tumour types have similar relations to host pigmentation characteristics (Beral et al. 1984).

Our results, showing an elevated risk of melanoma in subjects who burn easily and have poor tanning ability, are consistent with previous studies (Beitner et al. 1981; Beral et al. 1983; Lancaster and Nelson 1957; MacKie and Aitchison 1982). However, we found that although sunburn history was initially associated with risk of melanoma, when the analysis was controlled for skin reaction to sunlight a history of severe sunburns was no longer significant. The implication was that actual sunburn occurrence was less important than host pigmentation characteristics associated with poor sun tolerance.

Similarly, although individuals who never acquire a tan have an elevated risk of melanoma, when the analysis is controlled for skin reaction to sunlight the association disappears. Sunburn history and suntan history appear to be independent, as even when each is controlled for the other, both demonstrate a significant relationship with melanoma risk. However, each factor loses importance when controlled for skin reaction to sunlight. The implication is that the factor contributing to the risk of melanoma is the subject's tendency to burn and inability to tan. Sunburn history may therefore be indicative of a disturbance or deficit in melanocyte number or function, and the avoidance of acute sunburn by individuals who have a tendency to sunburn may not, therefore, reduce risk of melanoma.

Studies of melanoma have indicated that there is a relationship between risk of melanoma and sunlight exposure (Elwood and Hislop 1982; Holman et al. 1983; Lew et al. 1983). However, in a previous study we found that incidence of melanoma per unit body surface area was as common on intermittently exposed body sites as on usually exposed sites (Elwood and Gallagher 1983). Thus it seemed unlikely that risk of melanoma was directly related to cumulative sunlight dose. In addition, it has been pointed out that there is a deficit of melanoma in outside workers and higher rates in upper socioeconomic groups (Lee and Strickland 1980). It has been suggested that the risk of superficial spreading and nodular melanoma on skin which is little exposed to the sun is increased by intermittent exposure to intense sunlight, whereas chronic sunlight has little effect on risk (Elwood and Hislop 1982; Holman et al. 1983), and our findings provide support for this hypothesis. Outdoor workers, with a great deal of chronic sunlight exposure through their work, had no significantly increased risk of melanoma.

Subjects exposed to vacation sunlight exposure which, by definition, is intermittent, showed an elevated risk of melanoma. In addition, subjects with moderate to high levels of outdoor recreational activity also demonstrated an elevated risk of melanoma. Thus, the results for the three types of sunlight exposure are consistent with the hypothesis that intermittent heavy exposure increases the risk of melanoma while long-term chronic exposure has no effect.

It should be noted that analysis of the three exposure types by sex produced some differences in results (Elwood et al. 1985a). Female subjects reported less variation in occupational exposure, and although the increased risk for melanoma at higher vacation and recreation sunlight exposure is present in both sexes, it is stronger in women. On formal testing the difference between the sexes was not statistically significant for any of the three types of exposure. It may be that the differences are a result of the accuracy with which male and female subjects respond to questions about their sunlight exposure. Further studies will be necessary to clarify this issue.

The controversy in the epidemiological literature in regard to melanoma and hormonal factors in female patients has centred to date on use by women of exogenous preparations such as oral contraceptives and menopausal oestrogens. Our study results demonstrate no relationship between the use of oral contraceptives and risk of melanoma. Nor was any association seen with menopausal oestrogens.

Several case reports have suggested that individuals exposed to sunlamps may incur an increased risk of melanoma (Brodthagen 1982; Retsas 1983). Our results show no elevated risk for sunlamp use in either sex, for any anatomical site. Sunlamp use in our study was moderate, and it may be that the relatively limited exposure was not enough to shown any effect, but nevertheless our findings do not support the notion of a relationship with melanoma risk.

Overall, no association was seen between prior acne and risk of melanoma for either sex. When results were reviewed by sex a suggestion of an increased risk was seen for males, although it was not statistically significant. A previous study by Beral et al. (1983) found a history of acne to be protective, but their study included only female subjects. Laboratory studies have indicated that for certain tumours, short-term maintenance of melanoma cultures in vitro may proceed more favourably in the presence of androgens (Flax et al. 1973; Rampen and Mulder 1980). Since acne vulgaris is a disease thought to be activated by androgens beginning at puberty (Krupp and Chatton 1982) the possible association between acne and melanoma in male subjects may deserve further study.

No association was seen between psoriasis and melanoma in the Western Canada study, although an elevated risk for female patients was seen in an Australian study (Beral et al. 1983). A detailed study by Alderson and Clarke (1983) reported no significantly increased incidence of skin cancer in patients with prior psoriasis, but did not separate cutaneous melanomas from other skin tumours.

Viral diseases were essentially unrelated to risk of melanoma, with the exception of rubella, which appeared to be slightly more frequent in female cases than controls. No corresponding increase was seen in males. Although some laboratory work has suggested the presence of virus particles in animal tumours (Ito and Mishima 1967) and human tumours (Balda et al. 1975), there seems to be little evidence that common acute viral infection predisposes to melanoma, and our finding for rubella may be an artefact due to multiple testing.

Williams and Horm (1977) demonstrated an association between melanoma and alcohol use in data from the Third National Cancer Survey (1977), but we found no association with total alcohol consumption. Further analysis by sex and by type of alcoholic beverage (beer, wine, spirits) also showed no association.

The lack of association between smoking and melanoma incidence mirrors findings from a recently completed Australian study (Holman 1982).

Our dietary frequency questionnaire was relatively brief but covered most of the major items in a "western" diet. The lack of association with any particular foodstuff suggests that diet is not likely to be a major factor in the aetiology of malignant melanoma. It is possible that our instruments were not sensitive enough to detect nutritional intake differences, but a more detailed dietary workup by Holman (1982) also revealed little evidence to implicate food consumption as a melanoma risk factor.

To date, the major findings of the Western Canada Melanoma Study relate to host factors and sunlight exposure. Significant independent predictors of risk for melanoma are hair and skin colour, childhood freckling and skin reaction to sunlight. History of sunburning and tanning does not appear to be significantly related to melanoma risk independent of skin reaction to sunlight.

There is evidence from our study that intermittent exposure to strong sunlight is more important in the aetiology of melanoma than chronic long-term exposure, although further studies are necessary to confirm this.

Finally, our study offers no support for the putative association between use of oral contraceptives and elevated risk of cutaneous melanoma.

Acknowledgements. This paper is presented on behalf of the Western Canada Melanoma Study. Participants include:
Co-ordinators: M. Grace,[1] H. Colls †, D. Robson,[2] S. Kemel,[3] C. Leinweber,[1] and J. Moody.[4]
Pathologists: A. Worth[4] and W. S. Wood[4]
Consultants: M. L. Jerry,[1] M. D. P. Rebbeck,[4] D. McLean,[4] and H. K. B. Silver[4]
Secretaries: K. Anderson,[4] S. Morton,[4] and J. van den Broek[4]
We are grateful to the referring dermatologists, interviewers and subjects for their time and effort.

References

Adam SA, Sheaves JK, Wright NH, Mosser G, Harris RW, Vessey VP (1981) A case-control study of the possible association between oral contraceptives and malignant melanoma. Br J Cancer 44: 45-50

Alderson MR, Clarke JA (1983) Cancer incidence in patients with psoriasis. Br J Cancer 47: 857-859

Bain C, Hennekens CH, Speizer FE, Rosner B, Willett W, Belanger C (1982) Oral contraceptive use and malignant melanoma. JNCI 68: 537-539

Balda BR, Hehlmann R, Cho JR, Spiegelman S (1975) Oncornavirus-like particles in human skin cancers. Proc Natl Acad Sci USA 72: 3697-3700

Beitner H, Ringborg U, Wennersten G, Lagerlof B (1981) Further evidence for increased light sensitivity in patients with malignant melanoma. Br J Dermatol 104: 289-294

Beral V, Ramcharan S, Faris R (1977) Malignant melanoma and oral contraceptive use among women in California. Br J Cancer 36: 804-809

Beral V, Evans S, Shaw H, Milton G (1983) Cutaneous factors related to risk of malignant melanoma. Br J Dermatol 109: 165-172

Beral V, Evans S, Shaw H, Milton G (1984) Oral contraceptive use and malignant melanoma in Australia. Br J Cancer 50: 681-685

Breslow NE, Day NE (1980) Statistical methods in cancer research, vol 1. The analysis of case control studies. IARC Sci Publ 32

Brodthagen H (1982) Malignant melanoma caused by UV - A suntan bed? Acta Derm Venereol (Stockh) 62: 356-357

Clark WH, Mihm MC (1969) Lentigo maligna and lentigo-maligna melanoma. Am J Pathol 55: 39-67

Elwood JM, Gallagher RP (1983) Site distribution of malignant melanoma. Can Med Assoc J 128: 1400-1404

Elwood JM, Hislop TG (1982) Solar radiation in the etiology of cutaneous melanoma in Caucasians. Natl Cancer Inst Monogr 62: 167-171

Elwood JM, Lee JAH (1974) Trends in mortality from primary tumours of the skin in Canada. Can Med Assoc J 110: 913-915

[1] Alberta Cancer Hospitals Board, Edmonton, Alberta, Canada
[2] Saskatchewan Cancer Foundation, Regina, Saskatchewan, Canada
[3] Manitoba Cancer Treatment & Research Foundation, Winnipeg, Manitoba, Canada
[4] Cancer Control Agency of British Columbia, Vancouver, B.C., Canada

Elwood JM, Gallagher RP, Hill GB, Spinelli JJ, Pearson JCG, Threlfall W (1984) Pigmentation and skin reaction to sun as risk factors for cutaneous melanoma. Western Canada Melanoma Study. Br Med J I: 99-102
Elwood JM, Gallagher RP, Hill GB, Pearson JCG (1985a) Cutaneous melanoma in relation to intermittent and constant sun exposure - The Western Canada Melanoma Study. Int J Cancer 35: 427-433
Elwood JM, Gallagher RP, Davison J, Hill GB (1985b) Sunburn, suntan, and risk of cutaneous malignant melanoma: Western Canada Melanoma Study. Br J Cancer 51: 543-549
Flax H, Salih H, Westbury G (1973) Hormone therapy in malignant melanoma. Lancet II: 147
Gallagher RP, Elwood JM, Hill GB, Coldman AJ, Threlfall WJ, Spinelli JJ (1985) Reproductive factors, oral contraceptives and risk of malignant melanoma: Western Canada melanoma study. Br J Cancer 52: 901-907
Gellin GA, Kopf AW, Garfinkel L (1969) Malignant melanoma: a controlled study of possibly associated factors. Arch Dermatol 99: 43-48
Helmrich S, Rosenberg L, Kaufman DW, Miller DR, Schottenfeld D, Stolley PD, Shapiro S (1984) Lack of an elevated risk of malignant melanoma in relation to oral contraceptive use. JNCI 72: 617-620
Holly EA, Weiss NS, Liff JM (1983) Cutaneous melanoma in relation to exogenous hormones and reproductive factors. JNCI 70: 827-831
Holman CDJ (1982) Risk factors in the causation of human malignant melanoma of the skin. Ph. D. Thesis, University of Western Australia, Perth, pp 418-423
Holman CD, Armstrong BK (1984a): Pigmentary traits, ethnic origin, benign nevi and family history as risk factors for cutaneous malignant melanoma. JNCI 72: 257-266
Holman CDJ, Armstrong BK (1984b) Cutaneous malignant melanoma and indicators of total accumulated exposure to the sun: an analysis separating histogenetic types. JNCI 73: 75-82
Holman CDJ, Armstrong BK, Heenan PJ (1983) A theory of the etiology and pathogenesis of human cutaneous malignant melanoma. JNCI 71: 651-656
Holman CDJ, Armstrong BK, Heenan PJ (1984) Cutaneous malignant melanoma in women: exogenous sex hormones and reproductive factors. Br J Cancer 50: 673-680
Ito R, Mishima Y (1967) Particles in the cisternae of the endoplasmic reticulum of Fortner's amelanotic and melanotic malignant melanoma. J Invest Dermatol 48: 268-272
Klepp O, Magnus K (1979) Some environmental and bodily characteristics of melanoma patients. A case-control study. Int J Cancer 23: 482-486
Kopf AW, Kripke ML, Stern RS (1984) Sun and malignant melanoma. J Am Acad Dermatol 11: 674-684
Krupp MA, Chatton MJ (1982) Current medical diagnosis and treatment 1982. Lange Medical, Los Altos, California, pp 50-51
Lancaster HO, Nelson J (1957) Sunlight as a cause of melanoma: a clinical survey. Med J Aust 1: 452-456
Lee JAH, Strickland D (1980) Malignant melanoma: social status and outdoor work. Br J Cancer 41: 757-763
Lew RA, Sober AJ, Cook N, Marvell R, Fitzpatrick TB (1983) Sun exposure habits in patients with cutaneous melanoma: a case-control study. J Dermatol Surg 9: 981-986
Little JH, Holt J, Davis N (1980) Changing epidemiology of malignant melanoma in Queensland. Med J Aust 1: 66-69
MacKie RM, Aitchison T (1982) Severe sunburn and subsequent risk of primary cutaneous malignant melanoma in Scotland. Br J Cancer 46: 955-960
McGovern VJ, Caldwell RA, Duncan CA, Finlay-Jones LR, Hardy EG, Hicks JD, Little JH, Quinn RL (1967) Moles and malignant melanoma: terminology and classification. Med J Aus I: 123-124
McGovern VJ, Shaw HM, Milton GW, Farago GA (1979) Is malignant melanoma arising in a Hutchinson's melanotic freckle a separate disease entity? Histopathology 4: 235-242
Magnus K (1977) Incidence of malignant melanoma in the five nordic countries. Int J Cancer 20: 477-486

Mantel N, Haenszel W (1959) Statistical aspects of the analysis of data from retrospective studies of disease. JNCI 22: 719–748

Muir CS, Nectoux J (1982) Time trends: malignant melanoma of the skin. In: Magnus K (Ed) Trends in cancer incidence: causes and implications. Hemisphere, New York, pp 365–388

Nicholls EM (1968) Genetic susceptibility and somatic mutation in the production of freckles, birthmarks and moles. Lancet I: 71–73

Rampen FHJ, Mulder JH (1980) Malignant melanoma: an androgen dependent tumour? Lancet I: 562

Retsas S (1983) Sun beds and melanoma. Br Med J 286: 892

Swerdlow AJ, English J, Mackie RM, O'Doherty CJ, Hunter JAA, Clark J (1984) Benign nevi associated with high risk of melanoma. Lancet II: 168

Waterhouse J, Muir C, Shanmugaratnam K, Powell J (1982) Cancer incidence in five continents, vol IV. IARC Sci Publ 42

Williams RR, Horm JJ (1977) Association of cancer sites with tobacco and alcohol consumption and socio-economic status of patients: interview study from the Third National Cancer Survey. JNCI 58: 525–547

Epidemiology of Malignant Melanoma: Pigmentary Traits, Ultraviolet Radiation, and the Identification of High-Risk Populations, ***

N. Dubin, M. Moseson, and B. S. Pasternack

Institute of Environmental Medicine, NYU Medical Center,
New York University Medical Center, 550 First Avenue, New York, NY 10016, USA

Introduction

We report on a case-control study begun in 1979 to identify factors responsible for the observed high incidence of malignant melanoma among Caucasians. Interview data were collected on a comprehensive set of risk factors, including pigmentary characteristics, ultraviolet light exposure, family history, reproductive factors, drug use, ethnicity, smoking and dietary history, and chemical exposures. Quantification of risk factors was emphasized, whereas previous case-control studies had relied on qualitative assessments of exposure. A profile of high-risk individuals was to be developed for the purpose of identifying a subpopulation at whom future monitoring for malignant melanoma could be directed. In this report we present results for a subset of the available risk factor data, including pigmentary traits, sun exposure, and family history variables. Because of current interest in the relationship between fluorescent light exposure and melanoma risk (Beral et al. 1982; Maxwell and Elwood 1983; Pasternack et al. 1983) we include these data as well. The remaining risk factors will be analyzed in detail in subsequent reports.

Methods

Study Design

The study incorporated data from a large series of malignant melanoma patients interviewed at New York University Medical Center between 1972 and 1982. Although these data were originally collected for clinical purposes, the interview included a thorough epidemiologic questionnaire regarding known incidence risk factors. The addition of a control series between 1979 and 1982 enabled us to perform a case-control study of malignant melanoma. The same original interview data were collected from controls as from the cases. Supplementary epidemiologic questions, emphasizing quantitative exposures and new hypotheses, were added to the interview for both cases and controls starting in 1979.

---

* This work was supported in part by Grant OH-00915 (to BSP) from the National Institute for Occupational Safety and Health, and Center Grants CA-16087 and CA-13343 from the National Cancer Institute and ES-00260 from the National Institute of Environmental Health Sciences

** *Abbreviations: RR,* relative risk(s); *CI,* confidence interval(s); χ^2, chi-square; *df,* degree(s) of freedom

Table 1. Year of initial diagnosis for melanoma patients (n=1132)

Year of initial diagnosis	No. of patients	Percentage
(Nov.) 1972–1973	93	8.2
1974	82	7.2
1975	96	8.5
1976	130	11.5
1977	172	15.2
1978	157	13.9
1979	172	15.2
1980	127	11.2
1981–1982 (Jan.)	103	9.1
All years	1132	100.0

Melanoma Cooperative Group Case Series

Patients entering University Hospital, Bellevue Hospital, or Manhatten Veterans Administration Hospital for treatment of newly diagnosed primary malignant melanoma were given an interview and physical examination by the current Melanoma Fellow. Any lesion not histopathologically confirmed to be melanoma was excluded from the clinical data base. During the case accrual period there were four fellows serving consecutive terms, each trained by his predecessor to standardize the interview procedure.

Between November 1972 and January 1982 the total accrual of cases was 1132. Table 1 shows the distribution of cases by year of diagnosis. More cases accrued per year during the period 1977–1979 than either before or after. The relatively fewer cases available from the early years of the clinical registry may reflect increasing diagnosis of melanoma at our institution or, alternatively, incomplete enrollment of available cases. There were also fewer cases interviewed per year during 1980 and thereafter, coinciding with the opening of the Day Surgery facility at our institution. The speed with which patients were treated at and released from Day Surgery precluded interview for this study. Consequently, approximately one-third of melanomas were unavailable to the study for the final 2 years.

A preliminary analysis of our data (Pasternack et al. 1983) yielded a significant positive association between malignant melanoma and fluorescent light exposure. Because of the public health significance of such a finding, we conducted a reliability study to confirm our interview assessment of fluorescent light exposure. The reliability study was conducted by means of mailed questionnaires sent to all cases and controls.

Controls

Potential controls were randomly chosen from among patients 20 years of age and older appearing for a first visit to the New York University Skin and Cancer Unit general skin clinic or a first reregistration after 2 years absence. Patients under 20 years of age were excluded. Restricting controls to patients appearing for first visits or reregistration was designed to eliminate biases due to the over-representation of long-term patients with chronic skin disease. Although it was not possible for the Melanoma Fellows to interview controls, each control interview followed the standardized procedure developed for cases. A total of 748 controls were interviewed between October 1979 and January 1982, approximately twice as many as there were concurrent cases.

An additional 426 skin clinic patients refused to participate as controls. For a random sample of 100 of these we obtained basic demographic data and dermatologic diagnoses from the clinic records. Those who refused to participate differed only negligibly with respect to age, sex, marital status, race, year of visit, or dermatologic diagnosis.

Exclusions

Of the total of 1132 potential cases, 29 were excluded because of one of the following: age less than 20 years or unknown (10), non-white race (6), or previous melanoma (13). Of 748 potential controls, 163 were excluded for reasons of age (1), race (79), previous melanoma (8), other previous skin cancer (35), other previous malignancy (18), or current diagnosis of cancer (22). After exclusions, 1103 valid cases and 585 valid controls remained.

Patient Characteristics

The age and sex distributions for cases and controls are given in Table 2. The mean age of controls (43.0 years) was substantially younger than that of cases (52.1 years). The sex distributions for the two groups were similar, each having a slight preponderance of women.

Table 2. Age and sex distribution for melanoma patients (n=1103) and controls (n=585)

	Melanoma patients		Controls	
	Number	Percent	Number	Percent
Age, years				
20–29	96	8.7	197	33.7
30–39	153	13.9	105	17.9
40–49	214	19.4	75	12.8
50–59	268	24.3	62	10.6
60–69	225	20.4	84	14.4
70+	147	13.3	62	10.6
Sex				
Male	537	48.7	265	45.3
Female	566	51.3	320	54.7

Table 3. Anatomic location of melanomas (n=1103)

Anatomic location	No. of patients	Percentage
Trunk	410	37.2
Lower limbs	306	27.7
Upper limbs	210	19.0
Head and neck	165	15.0
Anogenital and crural	11	1.0
Unknown primary	1	0.1

With respect to the anatomic site of melanoma, nearly 40% of lesions were diagnosed on the trunk, more than one-quarter on the lower limbs, almost one-fifth on the upper limbs, and 15% on the head and neck (Table 3).

Pathological characteristics of the melanoma cases are given in Table 4. Nearly three-quarters were of the superficial spreading type; the only other sizable classification was nodular melanoma, diagnosed in under 10% of patients. Approximately one-half of patients included in the study were diagnosed at level IV or V. Accordingly, almost 60% had lesions thicker than 1 mm. Current dermatologic diagnoses of controls are given in Table 5.

There are more diagnoses than controls because as many as four diagnoses were recorded for each control. These represent a wide variety of skin conditions, with no single type of diagnosis predominant.

Assembly of Interview Data

Because of the study design, not all risk factor data are available for all subjects. Data on risk factors included in the original interview were obtained for all valid participants (1103 cases and 585 controls). Supplementary questions were added to the interview when we began to accrue controls. No attempt was made at that time to contact previously interviewed cases for these additional data. The supplementary interview questions were introduced at different times. Average hours per day of sun and fluorescent light exposure and

Table 4. Pathological characteristics of melanoma patients ($n = 1103$)

	No. of patients	Percentage
Histological type		
Lentigo maligna melanoma	52	4.7
Superficial spreading melanoma	813	73.7
Nodular melanoma	102	9.3
Acral lentiginous melanoma	35	3.2
Unclassified radial growth phase	50	4.5
Other	34	3.1
Unknown	17	1.5
Level of invasion		
I	43	3.9
II	250	22.7
III	265	24.0
IV	473	42.9
V	54	4.9
Unknown	18	1.6
Greatest thickness of lesion		
1.00 mm or less	456	41.4
1.01-2.00 mm	286	25.9
2.01-3.00 mm	133	12.1
3.01-5.00 mm	127	11.5
5.01-14.00 mm	72	6.5
Unknown	29	2.6

Table 5. Current dermatologic diagnoses of controls ($n=585$)

	Controls[a]	
	Number	Percent
Diagnosis		
Skin infections	57	9.7
Other infectious and parasitic diseases	84	14.4
Allergic diseases (internal agents)	18	3.1
Seborrheic dermatitis	43	7.4
Eczema	41	7.0
Contact and radiation dermatitis	38	6.5
Psoriasis and other scaling dermatoses	53	9.1
Pruritis and related conditions	42	7.2
Diseases of the nail, hair, hair follicles, and sweat and sebaceous glands	145	24.8
Nonmalignant neoplasms	164	28.0
Miscellaneous conditions[b]	125	21.4
Unknown	7	1.2

[a] Numbers do not total 585 and percentages do not total 100.0 because of multiple diagnoses among controls

[b] Includes hypertrophic and atrophic conditions, lichen planus, erythematous conditions, pilonidal cyst, insect bite, diseases of the circulatory system, dermatitis NOS, and other conditions diagnosed among fewer than ten patients

distribution of moles (Fig. 1) were asked of 289 cases and 585 controls. Skin color was assessed by means of the Scotto-Fears chart (Scotto and Fears 1978) for 472 cases and 585 controls. The freckling diagram (Fig. 2) was introduced last, yielding data on 208 cases and 457 controls.

All patients were given a physical examination during which the Melanoma Fellow counted the patient's moles and freckles. The mole and freckling diagrams were introduced because it proved impractical to undertake a physical examination of controls. Instead, controls were shown the diagrams (Figs. 1 and 2) and asked which most closely depicted their own mole and freckling distributions. Newly accruing patients were also shown the diagrams. For this subset of cases both the physician's count and the subject's own assessment could be compared. The concordance for moles was high: for 88.5% of subjects the categorization was identical by either method; the gamma statistic was 0.98 (Mueller et al. 1970). For this reasons we felt justified in combining the two mole counts as follows: the subject's own assessment was preferred, but when this was unavailable the physician's count was used. Unfortunately, such concordance was not achieved for degree of freckling; only 79.6% had identical categorizations, with a gamma of 0.94, so that we decided not to combine freckling data.

Reliability Study

The self-administered reliability questionnaire was mailed to all cases and controls between March and September of 1983. It consisted of quantitative questions on fluorescent light and sun exposure, as well as skin color. Skin color was included because we did not have a uniform assessment of it for all cases. Exposure data were related to the same time

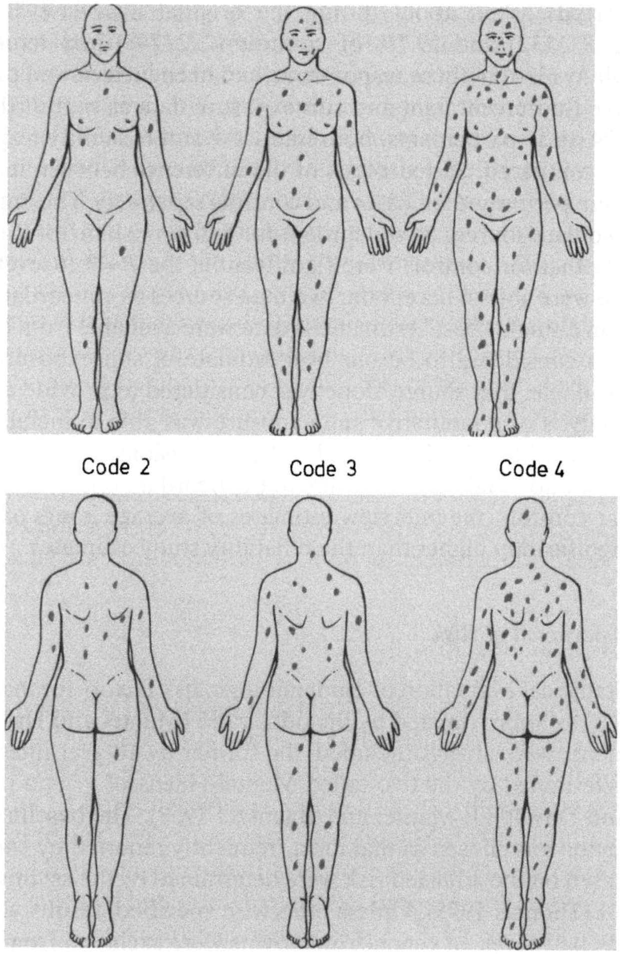

Fig. 1. Chart used for subjects' self-assessment of mole distribution

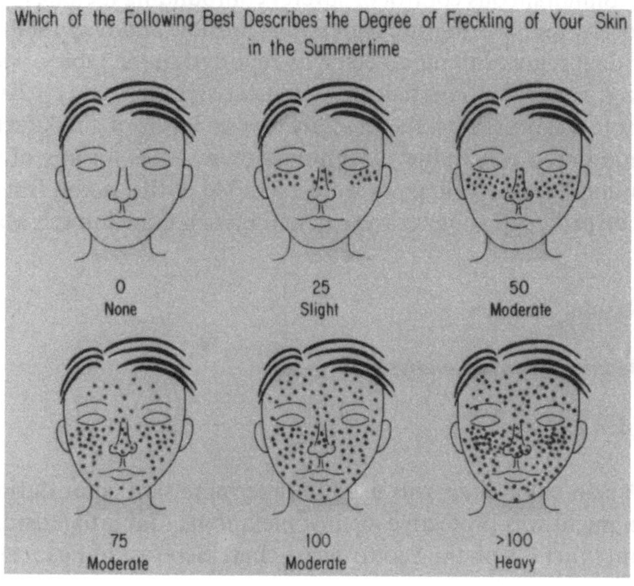

Fig. 2. Freckling diagram used for subjects' self-assessment of freckle pattern

periods asked about during the original interview. By March 1984, 44.9% of cases (508/1132) and 29.7% of controls (222/748) had returned completed questionnaires. Many (336) of these respondents had been interviewed prior to the collection of quantitative fluorescent light and sun exposure data as part of the supplementary interview. For 394 study participants, both interview and reliability responses were obtained and could be compared. Paired *t*-tests of the difference between interview and reliability responses were performed for cases and controls separately. The approach we took was to accept the two data sources as concordant for a given risk factor if neither the paired *t*-test for cases nor that for controls were significant at the $P=0.10$ level (two-tailed). For sun exposure, we were able to accept the two data sources as concordant and combined them as follows into a single "best" estimate: if data were available from both sources, the mean of the two was considered to be our best estimate of sun exposure; if only one data source were available, that source alone was considered to provide our best estimate. As a result, the analysis of quantitative sun exposure was able to include as many as 623 valid cases, as well as the 585 valid controls (after exclusions). For fluorescent light exposure the interview and reliability data were not concordant and were not combined. For cases, but not for controls, the interview estimates of average hours of fluorescent light exposure were significantly higher than the reliability study estimates.

Assessment of Risk

Statistical evaluation of epidemiologic risk factors for malignant melanoma employed the RR, as approximated by the odds ratio (Mantel and Haenszel 1959). Age and sex adjustments were always included, the former by 10-year intervals. Statistical significance was determined by the two-tailed Mantel-Haenszel χ^2 and pertinent tests for trend (Breslow and Day 1980; Mantel and Haenszel 1959). The baseline exposure group for each study factor was chosen as that most frequently reported by controls. Confidence intervals (CI) based on the adjusted risk were determined by the asymptotic maximum likelihood method (Thomas 1975). Unless otherwise specified, results were considered significant at the $P<0.05$ level. In general, unknowns were excluded from the analysis.

Simultaneous control of several confounding factors, in addition to age and sex, was effect by multiple logistic regression (Breslow and Day 1980). Statistical significance of individual regression parameters, as reported in the tables, was determined by the standardized regression coefficient. Statistical significance ($P<0.05$) for adding to or removing from a given model the possibly several levels of a risk factor was derived from the likelihood ratio test. Subjects with unknown values for any of the risk factors included in the multiple logistic analysis were excluded at this point, leaving 485 cases and 450 controls. The excluded subjects were nonetheless retained in the Mantel-Haenszel analysis.

Results

Mantel-Haenszel Analysis

Skin Color

A skin color chart was used to determine skin color during an interview. Increased skin pigment was protective against melanoma (Table 6) (trend, $P<0.05$). Subjects with medium skin (4-8 on the Scotto-Fears chart [Scotto and Fears 1978]) had 67% of the melanoma

Table 6. Relative risk of melanoma by skin characteristics

Risk factor	No. of melanoma patients[b]	No. of controls[c]	Mantel-Haenszel RR[d]	95% CI	Multiple logistic RR[e]
Skin color					
Pale[a]	409	455	1.00	-	
Medium	59	106	0.67*	0.46- 1.00	
Dark	2	12	0.30	0.04- 1.65	
Ability to tan					
None	114	41	1.53*	1.00- 2.44	2.39*
Light	328	127	1.46**	1.10- 1.95	1.49
Average[a]	456	247	1.00	-	1.00
Dark	185	166	0.58**	0.43- 0.77	0.67
Tendency to burn					
None	98	47	1.43	0.92- 2.19	3.90**
Mild redness only	271	135	1.19	0.89- 1.60	1.75*
Moderate burn	343	161	1.37*	1.04- 1.81	1.86**
Painful burn[a]	369	233	1.00	-	1.00
History of freckling					
No[a]	403	438	1.00	-	1.00
Yes	694	135	5.80**	4.50- 7.48	3.61**
Degree of freckling					
None to slight[a]	123	407	1.00	-	
Moderate	40	54	2.77**	1.64- 4.84	
Heavy	41	9	20.05**	8.09-54.04	
Mole count					
None	30	90	0.18**	0.10- 0.25	0.07**
1-25[a]	781	400	1.00	-	1.00
26-100	206	70	1.98**	1.41- 2.82	1.94**
>100	73	15	3.43**	1.85- 7.03	3.67**

[a] Baseline

[b] $n=1103$ for all factors except skin color ($n=472$) and degree of freckling ($n=208$) before exclusion of unknowns

[c] $n=585$ for all factors except degree of freckling ($n=457$) before exclusion of unknowns

[d] Adjusted for age and sex. Linear trend: Skin color, $P<0.05$; ability to tan, $P<0.0001$; tendency to burn, not significant; degree of freckling, $P<0.0001$; mole count, $P<0.0001$

[e] Adjusted for all other variables in the final multiple logistic model (see text)

* $P<0.05$; ** $P<0.01$

risk of subject with pale skin (9-10 on the chart). Those with dark skin (1-3 on the chart) had only 30% of the risk of those with pale skin. Results were very similar when we used the subjective determination from the mailed reliability questionnaire: "What is the color of your skin on a part of your body which is never exposed to the sun, such as under your arm or your buttocks? Compare your skin color with that of all races." The RR for those with medium skin was 0.76 and the RR for those with dark skin was 0.36 compared with those with pale skin (trend, $P=0.09$) (results not shown).

Ability to Tan

"Over the summer with gradual exposure, would you develop a tan that you would consider average for your basic skin color, or lighter or darker than average?" As can be seen from Table 6, the ability to tan is a protective factor ($P < 0.0001$); subjects who report a darker than average tan have half the risk (RR = 0.58) of those reporting average tanning ability, whereas those reporting no tanning or light tanning are at 50% increased risk (RR = 1.53 and RR = 1.46, respectively).

Tendency to Burn

"If you went out into the sun on a sunny summer day and stayed out two or three hours, what would happen to the previously unexposed parts of your body?" There was a 40% increased risk associated with either moderate or no tendency to burn as compared with painful burn (Table 6). Although the individual RR for moderate burn was significant, the overall tests of significance (global or trend) were not.

History of Freckling

"Freckles are brown spots which come and go with sun exposure. Do you get freckles now or did you as a child?" History of freckling was significantly associated with an almost sixfold risk of malignant melanoma (RR = 5.80; $P < 0.01$) (Table 6). The subjects' self-characterization of their current degree of freckling by means of Fig. 2 yielded a significant trend ($P < 0.0001$) toward increasing risk with increasing degree of freckling. As compared with those who do not freckle or freckle only slightly, moderate freckling had an RR of 2.77 ($P < 0.01$) and heavy freckling had an RR of 20.05 ($P < 0.01$). When we considered degree of childhood freckling the results changed only negligibly (not shown).

Mole Count

"Moles are spots which do not come and go with sun exposure. Some moles are flat, some are flesh-colored, and some have hair growing through them. What is the approximate number of moles that you have on your body (Fig. 1)?" The risk of melanoma increased significantly with increasing number of moles (trend, $P > 0.0001$) (Table 6). An absence of moles was protective (RR = 0.18, $P < 0.01$) compared with the baseline group (1-25 moles). There was an excess risk associated with reporting of more than 25 moles: a twofold risk (RR = 1.98, $P > 0.01$) among those reporting 26-100 moles, and a more than threefold risk (RR = 3.43, $P < 0.01$) among those reporting more than 100 moles.

Hair Color

"What was the natural color of your hair during the winter when you were twenty-five years old?" The melanoma risk associated with having red hair was more than five times (RR = 5.50, $P < 0.01$) that associated with having dark brown hair (Table 7). Neither blond

Table 7. Relative risk of melanoma by hair and eye color

Risk factor	No. of melanoma patients[b]	No. of controls[c]	Mantel-Haenszel RR[d]	95% CI	Multiple logistic RR[e]
Hair color					
Red	120	12	5.50*	3.16–12.74	2.16
Blond	160	72	1.27	0.89– 1.84	
Light brown	279	159	0.95	0.72– 1.26	1.00
Dark brown[a]	475	259	1.00	-	
Black	63	74	0.36*	0.23– 0.54	0.37*
Eye color					
Blue	425	85	3.07*	2.32– 4.26	2.56*
Green-gray-hazel	217	193	0.77	0.59– 1.01	1.00
Brown[a]	456	296	1.00	-	

[a] Baseline
[b] $n = 1103$ before exclusion of unknowns
[c] $n = 585$ before exclusion of unknowns
[d] Adjusted for age and sex
[e] Adjusted for all other variables in the final multiple logistic model (see text)
* $P < 0.01$

nor light brown hair was associated with a significantly different risk from dark brown hair. Those with black hair, however, had a significantly lower risk (RR=0.36, $P<0.01$) than those with dark brown hair.

Eye Color

Interviewer's observations of eye color were recorded. Subjects with blue eyes had three times the risk (RR=3.07, $P<0.01$) of subjects with brown eyes, whereas subjects with gray, green, or hazel eyes did not have a significantly different risk from brown-eyed subjects (Table 7).

Occupation Type

"Was your dominant lifetime occupation mostly indoors, mostly outdoors or both indoors and outdoors?" Compared with mostly indoor work, mostly outdoor work was associated with a more than doubled risk (RR=2.47, $P<0.01$) (Table 8). A lifetime work history that was half indoors and half outdoors carried no excess risk compared with mostly indoor work.

Recreation Type

"During most of your life, have you spent your free time mostly indoors, mostly outdoors or half indoors, half outdoors?" Subjects reporting mostly outdoor recreation had

Table 8. Relative risk of melanoma by qualitative sun exposure assessment

Risk factor	No. of melanoma patients[b]	No. of controls[c]	Mantel-Haenszel RR[d]	95% CI	Multiple logistic RR[e]
Occupation type					
Mostly indoors[a]	915	514	1.00	-	1.00
Both indoors and outdoors	87	51	1.04	0.69- 1.57	0.78
Mostly outdoors	94	20	2.47*	1.43- 4.36	2.43*
Recreation type					
Mostly indoors[a]	397	189	1.00	-	1.00
Both indoors and outdoors	322	285	0.59**	0.45- 0.76	0.55**
Mostly outdoors	372	110	1.65**	1.22- 2.25	1.03
Overall sun exposure					
None to little[a]	257	148	1.00	-	
Moderate	572	283	1.26	0.96- 1.67	
Much	258	143	1.13	0.82- 1.58	
Solar keratosis					
No[a]	984	560	1.00		1.00
Yes	110	9	5.04**	2.30-10.46	4.69**

[a] Baseline
[b] $n = 1103$ before exclusion of unknowns
[c] $n = 585$ before exclusion of unknowns
[d] Adjusted for age and sex. Linear trend: Occupation type, $P < 0.005$; recreation type, $P < 0.005$; overall sun exposure, not significant
[e] Adjusted for all other variables in the final multiple logistic model (see text)
* $P < 0.05$; ** $P < 0.01$

1.65 times the risk ($P < 0.01$) of subjects who spent their free time mostly indoors. A balance of indoor and outdoor recreation, however, afforded significant protection (RR = 0.59, $P < 0.01$) compared with mostly indoor recreation.

Overall Qualitative Sun Exposure

"In the course of your entire life, taking into consideration variation during different periods of time, would you say that you have gotten an average amount of sun exposure as compared to other people, or more or less than average?" As can be seen in Table 8, this variable was not a significant determinant of melanoma risk.

Solar Keratosis

The previous medical history was examined, and subjects reporting a previous history of solar keratosis had a fivefold risk of melanoma (RR = 5.04, $P < 0.01$) (Table 8).

Table 9. Relative risk of melanoma by quantitative sun exposure assessment (interview and reliability data combined)

Risk factor	No. of melanoma patients[b]	No. of controls[c]	Mantel-Haenszel RR[d]	95% CI
Sun exposure 0-5 years ago (h/day)				
0-1	218	166	1.22	0.89-1.68
2[a]	189	212	1.00	-
3	86	117	0.94	0.63-1.41
4	43	47	1.16	0.68-2.01
5+	34	38	1.10	0.58-2.07
Sun exposure 6-10 years ago (h/day)				
0-1	186	146	1.02	0.73-1.42
2[a]	191	185	1.00	-
3	100	118	1.08	0.73-1.61
4	49	67	0.97	0.59-1.60
5+	37	52	1.01	0.56-1.82
Sun exposure 11-20 years ago (h/day)				
0-1	154	103	0.98	0.68-1.42
2[a]	185	140	1.00	-
3	90	135	0.63*	0.41-0.92
4	70	92	0.74	0.47-1.16
5+	62	82	0.85	0.53-1.36

[a] Baseline
[b] $n=623$ before exclusion of unknowns
[c] $n=585$ before exclusion of unknowns
[d] Adjusted for age and sex. Linear trend: Sun exposure 0-5 years ago, not significant; sun exposure 6-10 years ago, not significant; sun exposure 11-20 years ago, not significant
* $P<0.05$

Quantitative Sun Exposure

Combined interview and reliability data were used. "What was the average number of hours spent in the sun per day during the last five years? Six to ten years ago? Eleven to twenty years ago?" Examination of Table 9 reveals no significant trends of increasing melanoma risk with increasing average hours of sun exposure during any of the three time periods of interest. When we examined the interview and reliability studies separately, similar results were found.

Quantitative Fluorescent Light Exposure

"What was the average number of hours spent under fluorescent light per day during the last five years? Six to ten years ago? Eleven to twenty years ago?" Examination of interview data showed a significantly increased risk among subjects reporting 7-8 average hours of exposure during the last 5 years (RR=3.07, $P<0.01$) and among those reporting

Table 10. Relative risk of melanoma by quantitative fluorescent light exposure (interview and reliability data separately)

Risk factor	No. of melanoma patients[b]	No. of controls[c]	Mantel-Haenszel RR[d]	95% CI
Interview				
Fluorescent light exposure 0-5 years ago (h/day)				
0-1	51	118	1.56	0.93-2.82
2-4	66	159	1.55	0.95-2.64
5-6[a]	52	167	1.00	-
7-8	77	82	3.07**	2.00-5.52
9+	16	33	2.30*	1.01-5.76
Reliability				
Fluorescent light exposure 0-5 years ago (h/day)				
0-1	134	49	1.37	0.85-2.28
2-4	106	47	1.09	0.66-1.82
5-6[a]	152	70	1.00	-
7-8	64	34	0.95	0.54-1.68
9+	23	19	0.61	0.28-1.29

[a] Baseline
[b] $n=289$ for interview and $n=506$ for reliability data before exclusion of unknowns
[c] $n=585$ for interview and $n=222$ for reliability data before exclusion of unknowns
[d] Adjusted for age and sex. Linear trend: Interview, not significant; reliability, not significant
* $P<0.05$; ** $P<0.01$

Table 11. Relative risk of melanoma by family history variables

Risk factor	No. of melanoma patients[b]	No. of controls[c]	Mantel-Haenszel RR[d]	95% CI
Melanoma in first-degree relative				
No[a]	1064	573	1.00	-
Yes	39	12	1.77	0.86-3.91
Other skin cancer in first-degree relative				
No[a]	993	543	1.00	-
Yes	110	42	1.37	0.92-2.10
Other malignancy in first-degree relative				
No[a]	684	426	1.00	
Yes	419	159	1.24	0.98-1.59

[a] Baseline
[b] $n=1103$
[c] $n=585$
[d] Adjusted for age and sex

9 hours or more on average of exposure during the last 5 years (RR = 2.30, $P < 0.05$) compared with those reporting an average exposure of 5-6 hours (Table 10). On the contrary, a weak, but nonsignificant, protective effect with increasing fluorescent light exposure was seen for the reliability study data. Although the results are not shown, the same pattern is repeated for exposure 6-10 years ago and 11-20 years ago.

Family History

Subjects' reports of melanoma, other skin cancer, or other malignancy in a parent, sibling, or offspring were recorded. Melanoma in a first-degree relative was associated with a nonsignificantly increased risk (RR = 1.77) (Table 11). Nonsignificant RR were also seen for a family history of other skin cancer and other malignancy.

Table 12. Relative risk of melanoma by weight, height, body mass index, and surface area

Risk factor	No. of melanoma patients[b]	No. of controls[c]	Mantel-Haenszel RR[d]	95% CI
Weight (lb)				
125 or less[a]	223	155	1.00	-
126-140	197	107	1.14	0.78-1.65
141-160	225	148	0.83	0.56-1.22
161-180	215	92	1.21	0.67-2.22
181 or more	219	74	1.13	0.63-2.12
Height (in.)				
62 or less	171	102	0.85	0.55-1.30
63-65	251	152	0.84	0.58-1.19
66-68[a]	270	158	1.00	-
69-71	218	109	1.24	0.86-1.81
72 or more	132	55	1.62*	1.01-2.65
Body mass index (lb/in.^{2})				
29 or less	177	128	1.20	0.82-1.76
30-32[a]	217	143	1.00	-
33-35	223	124	1.07	0.75-1.53
36-39	255	105	1.09	0.75-1.58
40 or more	168	75	1.01	0.68-1.51
Surface area (m^2)				
1.59 or less	207	126	1.14	0.75-1.74
1.60-1.71	191	130	1.02	0.70-1.48
1.72-1.85[a]	195	140	1.00	-
1.86-1.99	232	98	1.69**	1.15-2.58
2.00 or more	215	81	1.77**	1.20-2.90

[a] Baseline
[b] $n = 1103$ before exclusion of unknowns
[c] $n = 585$ before exclusion of unknowns
[d] Adjusted for age and sex. Linear trend: Weight, not significant; height, $P < 0.005$; body mass index, not significant; surface area, $P < 0.05$
* $P < 0.05$; ** $P < 0.01$

Table 13. Relative risk of melanoma by marital status

Marital status	No. of melanoma patients[b]	No. of controls[c]	Mantel-Haenszel RR[d]	95% CI	Multiple logistic RR[e]
Never married	138	233	0.36*	0.27–0.49	0.25*
Married[a]	749	261	1.00	-	1.00
Separated/divorced	49	54	0.36*	0.23–0.56	0.24*
Widowed	90	35	1.01	0.61–1.67	0.57

[a] Baseline
[b] $n = 1103$ before exclusion of unknowns
[c] $n = 585$ before exclusion of unknowns
[d] Adjusted for age and sex
[e] Adjusted for all other variables in the final multiple logistic model (see text)
* $P < 0.01$

Weight, Height, Body Mass, and Surface Area

As can be seen from Table 12, neither weight or body mass index (1000 times weight/height^2) was associated with melanoma risk. However, there was an increasing linear trend in melanoma risk for increasing height ($P < 0.005$). Surface area [$0.00718 \times \text{weight}^{0.425} \times \text{height}^{0.725}$ (Guyton 1976)] was also significantly associated with the risk of melanoma; subjects with a surface area of 1.86 m^2 or greater had approximately a 70% excess risk ($P < 0.01$) compared with subjects in the baseline group (1.72–1.85 m^2).

Marital Status

Unmarried subjects, whether never married, separated or divorced, had a decreased risk as compared to married subjects (RR = 0.36, $P < 0.01$) (Table 13). Widowed subjects had the same risk as married subjects.

Multiple Logistic Analysis

As many as possible of the variables considered in the Mantel-Haenszel analysis were retained in the multiple logistic analysis. Unfortunately, data based on the freckling diagram were available for relatively few participants; therefore, to maintain an adequate sample size we included only the dichotomous variable for history of freckling, which was recorded for all subjects. Skin color determined from the Scotto-Fears chart (Scotto and Fears 1978) was likewise available only for a relatively small proportion of the multiple logistic subset, which precluded its use here. Skin color as recorded on the reliability questionnaire was more widely available for this subset, but preliminary multiple logistic analysis indicated that this measure of skin pigment did not contribute significantly to the model after inclusion of the remaining skin characteristics listed in Table 6. Consequently, skin color was omitted from the subsequent multiple logistic analysis. Quantitative sun exposure was represented by the combined estimates of interview and reliability data. Fluorescent light exposure was excluded because of the observed discordance between the two data sources. Weight, height, and body mass index were omitted; of this grouping only surface area was included. All other variables were retained in the multiple logistic analysis; the categorical formats given in Tables 6 through 13 were used throughout.

Because this part of the analysis was based only on the subset of 485 cases and 450 controls with no missing data, it is pertinent to evaluate age- and sex-adjusted odds ratios for individual risk factors for this subset. In this way we could identify differences between this subset and the entire study group prior to the assessment of multiple risk factors simultaneously. There were few notable changes. The RR for red hair, as against dark brown hair, fell from 5.50 to 3.84; that for green, gray or hazel eyes, as against brown eyes, rose from 0.77 to 1.17. With respect to skin characteristics, for history of freckling the RR changed from 5.80 to 4.71, and that for no ability to tan, as against average ability to tan, rose from 1.53 to 1.87. Among qualitative sun exposure variables the RR for mostly outdoor work history, as against mostly indoor work history, fell from 2.47 to 1.82 and that for solar keratosis increased from 5.04 to 6.20. These RR modifications were due solely to the subset of patients available for the multiple logistic analysis, rather than to removal of the confounding effects of variables other than age and sex.

To examine the effects of multiple risk factors simultaneously, the variable selection procedure we used was to add a related group of risk factors to the model in a single step, followed by backward elimination of extraneous factors. The first step was to introduce all the skin characteristics (ability to tan, tendency to burn, history of freckling and the mole count), plus age (in 10-year intervals) and sex. A significant decrease in log-likelihood would have resulted from the removal of ability to tan ($\chi^2=24.2$, 3 *d.f.*, $P<0.005$), tendency to burn ($\chi^2=17.1$, 3 *d.f.*, $P<0.005$), or freckling ($\chi^2=72.4$, 3 *d.f.*, $P<0.005$), so that all were retained in the model. Next, hair color and eye color were added. Removal of blond and light brown hair from the model was not significant ($\chi^2=5.80$, 2 *d.f.*), nor was the removal of the indicator variable for green, gray, or hazel eyes ($\chi^2=0.05$, 1 *d.f.*). Indicator variables for red hair, black hair, and blue eyes were significant and were retained in the model along with all the skin characteristics. These formed a pigmentary group to which we added all qualitative and quantitative sun exposure variables. The quantitative sun exposure variable did not make a significant contribution to the log-likelihood ($\chi^2=3.49$, 2 *d.f.*). Solar keratosis, occupational sun exposure, and recreational sun exposure were significant and retained in the model, along with the pigmentary group, age and sex. Addition of the family history variables ($\chi^2=4.54$, 3 *d.f.*) or the surface area ($\chi^2=4.59$, 3 *d.f.*) was not significant. The addition of marital status, however, was significant ($\chi^2=44.8$, 3 *d.f.*, $P<0.005$). Our final multiple logistic model consisted of pigmentary variables (ability to tan, tendency to burn, freckling, mole count, red hair, black hair, and blue eyes), qualitative sun exposure variables (solar keratosis, occupational sun exposure, and recreational sun exposure), and marital status. RR from this final model are given in the far-right column in Tables 6, 7, 8, and 13. Compared with the Mantel-Haenszel analysis, multiple logistic RR differed substantially with respect to ability to tan (none, RR = 2.39), tendency to burn (none, RR = 3.90; mild redness only, RR = 1.75; and moderate burn, RR = 1.86), history of freckling (RR = 3.61), red hair (RR = 2.16), and mostly outdoor recreational exposure (RR = 1.03).

Discussion

Integration of Findings

Among the skin characteristics examined, freckling, particularly heavy freckling, number of moles, ability to tan, and tendency to burn were all significantly associated with the risk of melanoma. Skin color per se was not as strongly associated with the risk of melanoma as the other factors, an observation which confirms the recent findings of Holman and Armstrong (1984). Heavy freckling (more than 100 facial freckles) was the strongest risk factor in the study, having a twentyfold risk. Our findings for freckling are stronger than those reported by others (Beral et al. 1983; Elwood et al. 1984; Klepp and Magnus 1979), who did not use a standardized assessment such as Fig. 2. Similarly, use of a standardized means of quantitative assessment of moles on the body (Fig. 1) revealed a threefold risk to be associated with having more than 100 moles compared with having from 1 to 25 moles. This and other recent studies using mole counts provide especially strong support for an etiologic association between nevi and malignant melanoma (Beral et al. 1983; Holman and Armstrong 1984; Lee 1982; Reynolds and Austin 1984). Of methodologic interest is that use of Fig. 1 gave results consistent with a dermatologist's physical assessment of the patient's moles.

As expected (Elwood et al. 1984; Gellin et al. 1969; Holman and Armstrong 1984; Lee 1982; Lew et al. 1983), the ability to tan was inversely related to melanoma risk. In our study the ability to achieve a dark tan was associated with a 33% decreased risk, whereas the absence of any tanning ability whatsoever was associated with double the risk of subjects who characterize their tanning ability as average. The strong association we found between melanoma and tendency to sunburn was the reverse of that usually reported (Elwood et al. 1984; Holman and Armstrong 1984; Lee 1982; Lew et al. 1983; Reynolds and Austin 1984). Increasing tendency to burn was protective, with those subjects reporting no tendency to burn at almost four times the risk of those experiencing painful burn. Those of our subjects with greater tendency to sunburn also tended to have had less sun exposure; however, adjustment for sun exposure variables in the multiple logistic model left the RR for tendency to sunburn unaffected.

Our results for hair color and eye color followed the expected relationship (Beral et al. 1983; Gellin et al. 1969; Holman and Armstrong 1984). Having red hair or having blue eyes was associated with a doubled risk, and having black hair was associated with a one-third risk. The drop in RR for red hair from 5.50 in the Mantel-Haenszel analysis may in part be explained by the subset of cases and controls used in the multiple logistic analysis; for this subset the age- and sex-adjusted RR for red hair was 3.84. This was probably due to interviewer bias, because patients interviewed in earlier, as against later years were more likely to be excluded from the multiple logistic analysis due to missing data and were also more likely to be coded as having red hair. Nonetheless, the additional fall in RR from 3.84 to 2.16 may be attributed to the correlation of red hair color with other risk factors, such as freckling.

Of the qualitative sun exposure variables, history of solar keratosis was the strongest risk determinant (RR = 4.69), a finding which has not previously been reported. Mostly outdoor work experience was positively associated with the risk of melanoma (RR = 2.43), although there is a lack of consensus in the literature regarding such exposure (Cooke 1984; Holman et al. 1980, 1983; Klepp and Magnus 1979; Lee 1982; Mackie and Aitchison 1982; Paffenbarger et al. 1978). With respect to recreational activities, we found a decreased risk associated with participation in mixed indoor and outdoor activities

(RR = 0.55). The subjective nature of these qualitative sun exposure assessments makes them susceptible to differences in meaning for individual respondents. For these reasons we undertook the quantitative assessment of sun exposure. However, the quantitative assessment of sun exposure history was not associated with melanoma risk. This suggests that occupational and recreational sun exposure, although more subjective and less precise, may be indicative of the pattern of sun exposure that causes melanoma. One possible explanation of our findings is that out quantitative sun exposure variables measured exposure of the subject rather than exposure of the subject's skin. The strong relationship with solar keratosis, which reflects long-term heavy exposure of the skin to sunlight, supports this explanation. Qualitative assessments of sun exposure may inherently reflect the degree of protective clothing. An alternative explanation is that recall of hours of sun exposure may be sufficiently poor to obscure any relationship which exists. Another alternative is that cumulative exposure is not important per se, but that bursts of sustained exposure are a key factor in the development of melanoma. The available literature generally confirms the absence of a straightforward relationship with cumulative sun exposure, but has provided no definitive answers to date (Cooke et al. 1984; Gellin et al. 1969; Holman et al. 1980, 1983; Klepp and Magnus 1979; Lee 1982; Lew et al. 1983; Mackie and Aitchison 1982).

Our discordant results for fluorescent light exposure are disturbing. The reliability study data clearly do not support either the interview data that formed the basis of our preliminary report (Pasternack et al. 1983) or the findings of Beral et al. (1982). Despite all our efforts to the contrary, interviewer bias may have affected our fluorescent light data. The mailed questionnaire would be free of interviewer bias, but would exacerbate recall bias and introduce bias due to self-selection of subjects returning the questionnaire. For those subjects for whom both sources of fluorescent light data were available the interview data appeared to represent an overestimate of exposure relative to the reliability data but only for patients. This would explain the observed discrepancy in RR in Table 10. Unfortunately, no definitive answer can be provided by our study. We must look to other studies in progress to confirm an association between fluorescent light exposure and malignant melanoma.

Generally, earlier studies have reported a strong familial association for melanoma (Holman and Armstrong 1984; Lee 1982). The present study found a statistically nonsignificant increase in risk (RR = 1.77). This suggests that family history is not as important a risk factor for melanoma in our population.

Bias Due to Questionable Subsets of Cases and Controls

Patients enrolled prior to 1979 were not interviewed concurrently with controls. If there had been changes over time in demographic or other features of the source population a temporal bias might have resulted. We examined this by repeating our final multiple logistic model with noncurrent cases excluded.

For solar keratosis the RR rose to 8.62. The risk associated with no ability to tan (RR = 3.86) and light tanning ability (RR = 2.05) also increased when early cases were excluded. The RR for history of freckling decreased in magnitude, to 2.14, as did those for tendency to burn (none, RR = 2.72; mild redness only, RR = 1.14; and moderate burn, RR = 1.36). Although these individual risks changed in magnitude, overall trends in risk nevertheless remained unchanged.

Another possible source of bias was the loss of early-stage melanomas treated in Day Surgery since 1980. Cases included in the study since 1980 were more likely to be male (54.7%, as against 47.2% before 1980) and to have thicker lesions (2.16 mm average, as against 1.86 mm average before 1980), but did not differ with respect to age, site, or histological type of melanoma. Unfortunately, risk factor analysis excluding cases interviewed since 1980 would have little validity, as this would result in exclusion of almost all cases interviewed concurrently with controls.

The inclusion of certain diagnostic categories of controls could have affected the assessment of risk associated with sun exposure. For example, patients with acne or psoriasis are likely to be encouraged to increase their exposure to the sun. If this has occurred prior to their interview, substantial bias in RR can result. Re-examination of the final multiple logistic model, after excluding controls diagnosed with acne or psoriasis, indicated that such bias, if present, was negligible.

We were also curious as to whether certain diagnostic categories of controls might contain an unusually high proportion of single men or women, which might explain the low RR observed for never married, separated, and divorced subjects. There was some variation in marital status by diagnostic category, but we found this variation did not noticeably affect the RR for marital status.

Identification of High-Risk Groups

It is appropriate to consider whether our findings enable us to define a high-risk subpopulation from which all, or at least many melanoma cases are derived. If this were so, diagnostic efforts could be directed at monitoring this high-risk population for early detection of melanoma, since it is not generally feasible to screen the entire general population. In order to use our study results to identify a high-risk group, we must assume that the controls were randomly selected from the same underlying population as the cases. We must also assume the validity of risk factors identified in our study. Although we have not been entirely able to discount potential sources of bias, the strength and plausibility of our findings overall argue that they are likely to represent real associations with the development of melanoma.

Given these assumptions, can one identify a 10% subset of our population to account for 90% of cases? 75% of cases? 50% of cases? Consider heavy freckling (Table 6). This risk factor is exhibited in 20.1% (41/204) of cases, but only 1.9% (9/470) of controls. On the other hand, a history of freckling was present in 63.3% (694/1097) of cases, but also 23.6% (135/573) of controls. Pale skin color accounts for 87.0% (409/470) of cases, but a large proportion of controls, 79,4% (455/573), as well. Suppose we wish to limit our screening efforts to 10% or less of the underlying population at risk. To delineate such a subpopulation we may combine individual risk factors, each accounting for a small proportion of controls and a larger proportion of cases. For the high-risk group defined as all patients with heavy freckling or solar keratosis, our data indicate that we can account for 32.0% (65/203) of cases while limiting our screening effort to only 3.6% (17/467) of the skin clinic population of whites aged 20 years and older. If we add patients with no ability to suntan we can account for 41.0% (82/200) of cases while screening only 8.6% (40/464) of the population. Many other such combinations are possible, their usefulness depending on resources available for screening and the project benefit of early detection.

References

Beral V, Evans S, Shaw H, Milton G (1982) Malignant melanoma and exposure to fluorescent lighting at work. Lancet 2: 290-292

Beral V, Evans S, Shaw H, Milton G (1983) Cutaneous factors related to the risk of malignant melanoma. Br J Dermatol 109: 165-172

Breslow NE, Day NE (1980) Statistical methods in cancer research, vol 1. The analysis of case-control studies. IARC 122-159

Breslow NE, Day NE (1980) Statistical methods in cancer research, vol 1. The analysis of case-control studies. IARC pp 192-246

Cooke KR, Skegg DCG, Fraser J (1984) Socio-economic status, indoor and outdoor work, and malignant melanoma. Int J Cancer 34: 57-62

Elwood JM, Gallagher RP, Hill GB, Spinelli JJ, Pearson JCG, Threlfall W (1984) Pigmentation and skin reaction to sun as risk factors for cutaneous melanoma: Western Canada Melanoma Study. Br Med J 288: 99-102

Gellin GA, Kopf AW, Garfinkel L (1969) Malignant melanoma. A controlled study of possibly associated factors. Arch Dermatol 99: 43-48

Guyton AC (1976) Textbook of medical physiology. Saunders, Philadelphia, pp 953-954

Holman CDJ, Armstrong BK (1984) Pigmentary traits, ethnic origin, benign nevi, and family history as risk factors for cutaneous malignant melanoma. JNCI 72: 257-266

Holman CDJ, Mulroney CD, Armstrong BK (1980) Epidemiology of pre-invasive and invasive malignant melanoma in Western Australia. Int J Cancer 25: 317-323

Holman CDJ, Armstrong BK, Heenan PJ (1983) A theory of the etiology and pathogenesis of human cutaneous malignant melanoma. JNCI 71: 651-656

Klepp O, Magnus K (1979) Some environmental and bodily characteristics of melanoma patients. A case-control study. Int J Cancer 23: 482-486

Lee JAH (1982) Melanoma and exposure to sunlight. Epidemiol Rev 4: 110-136

Lew RA, Sober AJ, Cook N, Marvell R, Fitzpatrick TB (1983) Sun exposure habits in patients with cutaneous melanoma: a case-control study. J Dermatol Surg Oncol 9: 981-986

Mackie RM, Aitchison T (1982) Severe sunburn and subsequent risk of primary cutaneous malignant melanoma in Scotland. Br J Cancer 46: 955-960

Mantel N, Haenszel W (1959) Statistical aspects of the analysis of data from retrospective studies of disease. J Natl Cancer Inst 22: 719-748

Maxwell KJ, Elwood JM (1983) UV radiation from fluorescent lights. Lancet 2: 579

Mueller J, Schuessler K, Costner H (1970) Statistical reasoning in sociology. Houghton Mifflin, Boston, pp 279-292

Paffenbarger RS Jr, Wing AL, Hyde RT (1978) Characteristics in youth predictive of adult-onset malignant lymphomas, melanomas, and leukemias: brief communication. JNCI 60: 89-92

Pasternack BS, Dubin N, Moseson M (1983) Malignant melanoma and exposure to fluorescent lighting at work. Lancet 1: 704

Reynolds P, Austin DF (1984) Epidemiologic-based screening strategies for malignant melanoma of the skin. In: Engstrom PF, Anderson PN, Mortenson LE (eds) Advances in cancer control: epidemiology and research. Liss, New York, pp 245-254

Scotto J, Fears TR (1978) Skin cancer epidemiology: Research needs. Natl Cancer Inst Monogr 50: 169-177

Thomas DG (1975) Exact and asymptotic methods for the combination of 2 × 2 tables. Comput Biomed Res 8: 423-446

*Risk Factors for Cutaneous Melanoma in Queensland**, **

A. Green, C. Bain, R. McLennan, and V. Siskind

Queensland Institute of Medical Research, Bramston Terrace, Herston, Brisbane 4006, Australia

Introduction

Both incidence and mortality rates of cutaneous melanoma appear to have increased over several decades in many populations. Incidence rates have increased rapidly (Elwood and Lee 1979) in culturally diverse, though largely pale-skinned, populations, especially for melanomas on the lower limbs of females, trunks of males, and upper limbs of both sexes. Mortality rates have risen 3% to 9% per year (Elwood and Lee 1979), and in successive birth cohorts. In Australia there is evidence that increased rates began in people born around 1865 (Armstrong et al. 1982).

Melanocyte density varies with different anatomical sites of the skin, increasing in density from trunk to extremities, head, and foreskin (Szabo 1967), with age (Gilchrest et al. 1979), and with exposure to ultraviolet radiation (UVR) (Quevedo et al. 1965). Certain benign proliferative melanocytic lesions have been associated with increased risk of melanoma: (a) *Lentigines,* which have hyperplasia of a single layer of melanocytes with hyperpigmentation of the basal layers of the epidermis and no increase in pigmentation after exposure to sunlight (freckles, in contrast, have a normal number of hyperpigmented melanocytes which darken after UVR exposure); and (b) *naevi* (moles), specifically in this study the common naevus, a benign tumour of melanocytes with both hyperplasia and multiple layers, present in varying numbers in most people, and appearing as tan to deep brown pigmented macules, papules or patches. The association between moles and melanomas is unclear, but approximately two-thirds to three-quarters of patients with melanoma report an antecedent lesion (Ariel 1980; McNeer and Gupta 1964), and 25%-50% have histological evidence of an associated naevus (Elder et al. 1980; McGovern 1977). The simplest explanation is that the cells of a naevus may undergo neoplastic transformation, as may any epidermal melanocyte (Clark et al. 1977).

Elder et al. (1982) view dysplasia in naevi as an evolutionary stage which may progress to an overtly neoplastic melanoma directly analogous to other sequential transformations

* The study described in this paper was supported by the National Health and Medical Research Council and the Queensland Cancer Fund. Assistance in contacting clinicians and pathologists was given by the Queensland Melanoma Project

** *Abbreviations: SSM,* superficial spreading melanoma; *LMM,* lentigo maligna; *NM,* nodular melanoma; *IND,* indeterminate melanoma; *ACL,* acral lentiginous melanoma; *OC,* oral contraceptive

Recent Results in Cancer Research. Vol 102

of precursor lesions, e.g., the development of invasive carcinoma in the head of a dysplastic adenomatous polyp of the colon. Alternatively, Happle et al. (1982) view naevi as phenotypic indicators of a hereditary disposition to cutaneous melanoma.

There is considerable evidence that exposure to UVR plays a major role in the aetiology of cutaneous melanoma. The quantity of terrestrial UVR depends on many factors - solar variability; variations in the sun-earth distance; absorption by molecules in the atmosphere, scattering by particles, such as dust, aerosols, water droplets (clouds), and other factors contributing to the turbidity of the atmosphere; absorption by ozone in the upper atmosphere; reflection from the clouds and lower atmosphere where UVR returns to earth as backscattering; and reflection from the earth's surface. Water reflects 4.5% of incident UVR, dry and wet sand reflect 12% and 8%, respectively, and the lowest reflectance comes from vegetation (green grass) with 1.5% (Barton and Paltridge 1979). The effects of high UVR exposure range from the acute sunburn reaction of the skin through the spectrum of chronic cutaneous damage. Sunburn in its mildest form consists of delayed erythema of the skin appearing 1-4 h after exposure and gradually fading after 1-3 days. Severe sunburn causes inflammation, blistering and peeling of the skin, with tanning perhaps noticeable within 2 or 3 days. Repeated sun exposure causes general degenerative changes in human skin comprising atrophy, freckling with hyper- and hypopigmentation, telangiectases, abnormal elastic tissue formation in the dermis with yellow discolouration, and manifest wrinkling. Chronic solar exposure results in actinic keratoses and malignant skin lesions (Pinkus 1976). There is extensive evidence for the causal role of sunlight in the production of nonmelanoma skin cancers (Forbes et al. 1979). Data on the measured UVR transmittance of human skin have been summarized by Daniels (1979), who concludes that in white skin there is significant transmission of sunburn radiation to the dermis. The melanin pigment produced by melanocytes filters the UVR incident on the skin, shielding the deeper layers of the epidermis and the dermis. In areas often exposed to the sun, abnormal forms are occasionally found which stain deeply after dopa reaction. These abnormal melanocytes are never found in unexposed sites, and are most abnormal where the dose of solar radiation had been very high and the protection from natural pigmentation low (Mitchell 1963). A numerical increase in epidermal melanocyte precursors follows repeated UVR exposure (Jimbow and Uesugi 1982). This may result from activation of melanocyte precursors and their mitotic proliferation, or from proliferation of melanocytes present prior to exposure (Rosdahl 1979; Rosdahl and Szabo 1978). In sites exposed to the sun, melanocytes are larger, and their processes particularly long in sites where melanocytes are infrequent, such as the leg (Mitchell 1963).

Lee (1982) has reviewed data relating melanoma to exposure to sunlight. The lentigo maligna (LMM) type is associated with cumulative UVR exposure, as was recognized in early descriptions of "la melanose circonscrite précancéreuse" in Bordeaux vineyard workers (Dubreuilh 1912) who typically had the advanced age and outdoor activities of LMM patients, and the exposed sites of the lesions. The epidemiology of LMM is thus similar to that of basal cell (BCC) and squamous cell carcinomas (SCC) of the skin, while the relation of the other types of melanoma to UVR requires more specific analytical studies than those done in the past, especially in relation to intermittent exposure to UVR. Because incidence rates of melanoma differ between women in reproductive life and men of the same ages (Lee and Storer 1980), and because there are data which suggest oestrogens and progestogens may stimulate melanocytes (Snell 1967), it has been proposed that melanoma in women is associated with various hormonal risk factors. Specific evidence of their importance as initiators or promoters of melanoma is lacking, however. Oestrogen receptors have been found in human melanoma cells (Chaudhuri et al. 1980), but their significance is questionable (Neilfield and Lippman 1980). Use of oral contraceptives (OCs) has been assessed in relation to a possible increase in risk, with mixed results (Adam et al. 1981; Bain et al. 1982; Beral et al. 1977; Helmrich et al. 1984). The effect of pregnancy is disputed (Shiu et al. 1976), while late age at first birth has recently been reported to increase risk (Holly et al. 1983). The possibility exists that results to date have been biased because of an absence of information about exposure to sunlight in the women investigated.

Various chemicals, diet, radiation and viruses have been suggested as risk factors (Farber 1981), in addition to or independent of ultraviolet radiation. Isolated reports have implicated various industrial exposures, based on extremely small numbers of cases (Lee 1982). Candidate exposures include that to polychlorinated biphenyls (Bahn et al. 1976); the occupational exposures of chemists (Hoar and Pell 1981; Thomas and Decoufle 1979) and of gold miners (Armstrong et al. 1979); arsenic (associated with skin cancer in factory workers (Clough 1980); diazepam (Horrobin and Troska 1981); and suntan preparations containing psoralens, since in the presence of UVR, melanogenesis is promoted by 5-methoxypsoralen, a compound mutagenic (Ashwood-Smith et al. 1980) and tumorigenic in mice exposed to UVR (Zajdela and Bisagni 1981). Endogenous topical skin agents from the photoproducts of cholesterol could also be implicated, e.g., cholesterol α-oxide, which results from acute or chronic exposure to UVR, is found in the serum of patients with elevated serum cholesterol, and has carcinogenic properties (Chan and Black 1976). Cholesterol α-oxide is a carcinogen, which may be formed after UVR exposure in mouse (Black and Douglas 1972) and human skin (Black and Lo 1971). Some topical products may screen the skin from UVR. Surface layers of dead cells contribute to the thickness of the stratum corneum which filters UVR (Daniels 1969); excessive washing may remove some of this natural protection (McCarthy 1981).

Williams (1976) suggested the possibility of a correlation between melanoma and alcohol consumption through promotional activity by alcohol-induced pituitary secretion of MSH. Overall, however, investigations into the role of dietary factors in the aetiology of melanoma have been few.

An excess of melanoma was found in the employees of Lawrence Livermore Laboratory in California engaged in high-energy (nuclear) physics research (Austin et al. 1981) but not in a comparable laboratory in New Mexico (Acquavella et al. 1982). In the initial California series the observed occupational risks appeared to be mediated by other determinants of susceptibility, namely a history of parental skin cancer, and presence of six or more moles greater than 0.5 cm in diameter (Reynolds et al. 1982). However, an elevated risk remained for the occupational grouping of "chemists". Another kind of radiation risk, exposure to fluorescent light sources, was suggested by Beral et al. (1982) based on a case-control study of a group of female melanoma patients in Sydney. However, the risk was confined to fluorescent exposure at work (particularly in offices) rather than at home, and the increased risk remains to be confirmed. Patients with malignant melanoma of the skin frequently report previous trauma at the site, both acute episodes and chronic irritation. Viruses have also been suggested as possible causative agents (Birkmayer et al. 1974; Parsons et al. 1976) through firm evidence is lacking.

Melanoma of all histological types has been described in families (Bork et al. 1981). They usually arise from the same organ, e.g., skin or eye (Miller and Pack 1962). Sensitivity to UVR has been studied in members of melanoma-prone families (Ramsay et al. 1982). Using lymphoblastoid cell lines, decreased cell survival after UVR irradiation indicated cell sensitivity. All patients with melanoma, and those with multiple naevi, were found to be UVR sensitive. The data appeared to be consistent with a dominantly inherited UVR light sensitivity.

The UVR dose to the melanocyte does not equate with the UVR exposure received at the skin surface, but is conditional on epidermal transmission. The following conceptual model is proposed:

UVR EXPOSURE AT SURFACE	minus	LOSS IN EPIDERMAL TRANSMISSION	equals	UVR DOSE TO MELANOCYTE

Thus a high level of sun exposure would result in a *maximum* UVR dosage when there was a high level of UVR in the ambient sunlight and when UVR loss in surface-to-melanocyte transmission was low; and in *low* dosage when there was a low level of UVR in the ambient sunlight and/or when there was a high loss of UVR during epidermal transmission. The amount lost in epidermal transmission depends on host factors which are largely under genetic and environmental control and which can be examined, e.g., inherent skin colour, propensity to sunburn, level of tanning, etc. In practical situations, a high cumulative UVR dose may be delivered to the melanocyte in peaks of UVR dosage at intervals, i.e., at high dose rates, or chronically over a long period, i.e., at low dose rates. Either method of accumulating high UVR might be consistent with a dose-dependent model of UVR carcinogenesis.

There is an interplay between genetic factors determining susceptibility to UVR and the UVR dose received. The susceptibility to carcinogenesis may be "general", as in a family history of various types of cancer, e.g., resulting from a defective immune surveillance. On the other hand, the genetic susceptibility may exist specifically at the level of the melanocyte, with some abnormality of the genome. For example, melanocytes comprising visible proliferative lesions like naevi or lentigine may be atypical compared with melanocytes which exist and function individually in the context of an epidermal melanin unit ("normal" melanocytes).

In terms of a multistage concept of carcinogenesis, melanocytes, atypical or normal, may first undergo initiation from a mutagenic effect of high UVR dose mediated by melanocyte susceptibility. Initiation could also occur spontaneously or as the result of other agents, such as X-radiation or chemical carcinogens. Promotion to overt neoplasia, i.e., beyond melanocytic dysplasia, could occur as a result of the action of such agents as chemicals or hormones or of further doses of UVR. Melanocytes liable to proliferation, either inherently (naeval or lentiginous cells) or as a function of previous exposure (e.g., extreme UVR stimulation), would be particularly susceptible to neoplastic change. It is postulated that some melanomas may not have a discernable dysplastic stage.

Methods

Cases

The data presented here were collected in the course of a case-control study of cutaneous malignant melanoma. Eligible case subjects were all persons resident in Queensland who had a first primary cutaneous melanoma reported at routine diagnosis by a pathologist in the year from 1 July, 1979 to 30 June 1980. No review of the histological findings was undertaken: melanoma is diagnosed relatively frequently in Queensland, and there is free exchange of problem slides between pathologists (Little et al. 1980). From a source population of 871 such cases, a random sample of 243 cases was drawn, stratified by geographical location of residence to ensure representation of cases from the less densely populated interior part of the State. In all, 236 patients (97% of the random sample) aged between 14 and 86 years were interviewed. The histological types were melanoma with adjacent component of superficial spreading type (SSM, 141 subjects); melanoma with adjacent component of lentigo maligna (LMM, 49); nodular melanoma (NM, 35); melanoma of indeterminate classification (IND, 7); and acral lentiginous melanoma (ACL, 4). LMM and ACL are considered aetiologically different subtypes (Feibleman et al. 1980; McGovern et al. 1980), and the analysis was generally restricted to the 183 cases of SSM, NM and IND types.

Controls

Each of the cases was matched with a control subject by age (within 5 years), sex, and location of residence in Queensland, controls being selected at random from the State electoral roll. The Australian Bureau of Statistics divides the State (1 727 000 km^2 in area) into 11 such statistical divisions (Green en Siskind 1983), and these were considered large enough to minimize the likelihood of geographical "overmatching" of subjects. Because enrolment is compulsory by law, the electoral roll sampling frame embraces virtually the whole of the adult population of Queensland. Excluding 13 persons who had moved from the addresses listed on the roll, the 236 controls represented 92% of the original community sample.

Interviews

All subjects were personally interviewed by one of us (AG). Most interviews were conducted in the subjects' homes, though a small number of subjects (both patients and controls) were visited at their place of work and 15% of patients and 3% of controls were interviewed in hospital out-patients' departments. A standard questionnaire was used and histories of lifetime sun exposure were obtained by documenting all outdoor occupations held for more than 6 months and all recreations ever pursued on a regular basis after 10 years of age. Total hours of sun exposure were estimated by summation of reported occupational and recreational sun hours for the whole of life (from 10 years of age); an estimate of total UVR exposure was derived from each subject's residential history with information on the average UVR level (Paltridge and Barton 1978; Schulze 1978). Respondents were asked to recall all episodes of severe sunburn where pain had persisted longer than 48 h, with or without blistering. The number of sunburn experiences (to a maximum of 9) was recorded by age group (0-9, 10-19, 20-29, 30+). All burns reported occurred before the age of 40 (except 5 in cases and 3 in controls). Other factors included the individual's complexion, sun sensitivity, hair colour at age 21 as graded against a standard colour chart, and propensity to sunburn in the standard situation of exposure to the sun for an hour for the first time.

Questions were also asked about social and personal factors which may relate to melanoma. Social class was ranked according to subjects' occupation, or in the case of dependants, on the occupation of the main income earner. Migrant status and ethnic background were based on subject's country of birth and those of parents and grandparents plus subject's age at migration.

Female respondents were asked about their menstrual and reproductive histories and their use of OCs and other hormonal preparations prior to the date of case diagnosis. As a further index of endogenous hormonal exposure, duration of ovulatory life in years was calculated. This was obtained by subtracting total years of OC use and an anovulatory year for each full-term pregnancy from total years between menarche and menopause (or current age if still menstruating).

Examination of the Skin

At the completion of interview the face and left forearm were examined. Actinic tumours were grouped on a continuum from solar keratoses to BCCs and SCCs, as these lesions when small are often indistinguishable clinically (Beardmore 1982). Solar keratoses were defined as reddened hyperkeratoses and were regarded as epidermal carcinoma in situ (Pinkus 1971). Typical BCCs were identified by their pearly edge or center, and SCCs often appeared redder, with a more crusted surface. The presence of sundry pigmented lesions, particularly pigmented naevi, on the left arm below the tip of the shoulder was also noted. Naevi were defined as dark brown (presumed melanocytic) lesions, 2 mm or greater in diameter and could be either macular or raised. The latter usually distorted the normal reticular pattern of the skin surface. In contrast, lentigines which were counted separately, were paler macular lesions. Large lentigines had irregularly crenated borders compared with the relatively smooth even if irregular, borders of naevi. No differentiation was made between types of common acquired naevi, e.g., junctional versus intradermal.

Analysis

The first stage of analysis used simple univariate screening, both matched and unmatched, to identify major crude associations. The strength of melanoma-exposure associations was measured by the exposure odds ratio, which approximates the relative risk (RR) (Cornfield 1951), and 95% confidence intervals were constructed to assess statistical significance. Stratified group-based analysis (ignoring the matching) comprised the next stage (Mantel and Haenszel 1959). Likely confounding variables were identified during this step, and effect modification and biological interrelationships were explored. Multivariate modelling with retention of the matching was applied to achieve a final estimate of risk with simultaneous control of extraneous factors. A conditional logistic model for matched pairs was used (Breslow and Day 1980).

An important measure of validity was an assessment of interviewer bias. While cases were known to have melanoma at interview, their specific histological type was not known. Subsequent data analysis revealed substantial differences with respect to sunburn exposure (Table 1) and the presence of both naevi and lentigine among LMM cases and other types, but not among their matched controls.

Results and Comment

Pigmentary Factors

The strongest association between melanoma and pigment phenotype was for the presence of proliferative lesions on the arms (Green et al. 1985a). Taking as standard the absence of the particular lesion from the arms, RRs for increasing numbers of lentigines

Table 1. Distribution of sunburn episodes among cases and controls by histological group of cases

Histological group	SSM, NM and IND			LMM		
	Cases	Controls	Crude RR[a]	Cases	Controls	Crude RR[a]
No. of subjects	183	183		49	49	
Sunburn episodes						
0–1	84	128	1.0	36	32	1.0
2–5	51	33	2.4	7	10	0.6
6+	48	22	3.3	6	7	0.8

[a] Relative risk calculated ignoring individual matching

Table 2. Propensity to proliferative melanocytic lesions on the arms and crude risk of melanoma

	None	Number of naevi on arms			Any
		2–4	5–10	>10	
Cases	29	93	44	17	154
Controls	137	28	14	4	46
Relative risk[a]	1.0	16.0	14.6	20.1	15.8 28.0[b]

	None	Number of lentigines on arms			Any
		2–4	5–10	>10	
Cases	47	44	41	51	136
Controls	122	22	19	20	61
Relative risk[a]	1.0	5.2	5.6	6.6	5.8 6.9[b]

[a] Relative risk calculated ignoring individual matching
[b] Relative risk taking account of individual matching

were 5.2 (1–4 lesions), 5.6 (5–10) and 6.6 (more than 10 lesions); the respective RRs for naevi on the arms were 16.0, 14.6 and 20.1 (Table 2). These data showed the major effect was the presence of any lesions, rather than a strong trend with increasing numbers of lesions. When taken as dichotomous exposures the RR for melanoma in the presence of lentigines was 5.8; and that in the presence of naevi 15.8 (with a matched estimate of 28.0–almost double the unmatched estimate in this one exceptional case). The presence of naevi was associated with the presence of lentigines. The RR of lentigines with naevi is 4.9 in cases and 4.3 among controls. The RR for melanoma associated with lentigines after adjustment for naevi was 2.7 (1.6–4.5). The RR when naevi were present after adjustment for lentigines was 11.2 (6.8–18.5). When both naevi and lentigines were present the RR for melanoma was 29.3 (1.62–53.1) compared with the absence of both.

Risk factors relating to cutaneous phenotype (Table 3) were also found to be crude predictors of risk of melanoma (Green et al. 1985a), the matched estimates of risk being generally similar to those obtained from unmatched analysis. Results after stratification of

Table 3. Constitutional and phenotypic characteristics and melanoma risk: crude and adjusted for presence of naevi and lentigines

	Cases	Controls	Crude RR[a]	Adjusted RR	
				For naevi	For lentigines[b]
Propensity to sunburn					
Tan only	12	31	1.0	1.0	1.0
Burn then tan	41	58	1.8	1.9 (0.7–5.0)	1.8 (0.8–4.2)
Burn then peel	130	94	3.6	2.5 (1.0–6.1)	3.8 (1.7–8.4)
Depth of tan					
Dark	33	68	1.0	1.0	1.0
Moderate	126	104	2.5	1.6 (1.1–2.4)	1.5 (0.9–2.7)
No tan	24	11	4.5	3.0 (1.1–8.1)	1.6 (0.6–4.5)
Ease of tanning					
Easily	65	97	1.0	1.0	1.0
Slowly	89	63	2.1	1.6 (0.9–2.8)	1.2 (0.7–2.0)
Not at all	29	23	1.9	1.0 (0.5–2.2)	0.8 (0.4–1.7)
Propensity to freckle					
Absent	97	137	1.0	1.0	1.0
Present	86	46	2.6	1.5 (0.9–2.5)	1.1 (0.6–1.9)
Hair colour					
Black/dark brown	22	47	1.0	1.0	1.0
Light brown/blonde	136	121	2.4	1.9 (1.0–3.6)	1.8 (0.8–4.2)
Red	25	15	3.6	2.4 (1.0–5.8)	3.8 (1.7–8.4)
Eye colour					
Brown	32	54	1.0	1.0	1.0
Blue/grey	95	82	2.0	2.4 (1.2–4.5)	1.3 (0.7–2.4)
Green/hazel	56	47	2.0	2.2 (1.1–4.5)	1.6 (0.8–2.9)
Skin colour (left forearm)					
Olive	32	48	1.0	1.0	1.0
Fair	151	135	1.7	1.0 (0.6–1.9)	0.9 (0.5–1.6)

[a] Relative risk calculated ignoring individual matching
[b] 95% confidence limits

inducible and inherent pigment data by the variables representing the presence of naevi and lentigines showed that most of the crude associations were reduced in strength to varying degrees (Table 3). The phenotypic characteristics in Tables 2 and 3 were coded into dichotomies, if necessary with the aid of dummy variables, and included in a conditional logistic model for matched pairs. The results are given in Table 4. In this analysis each risk factor is adjusted for the present of all others. The strongest association was found between melanoma and naevi on the arms (RR of 22.8); that for the simpler proliferative disorder lentigines on the arms was much less (2.7). Other strong associations were propensity to sunburn with or without peeling (5.0) and hair colour (light brown or blonde 3.8; red 7.2). There was no evidence that patients with naevi had different types of tumour from those without naevi. The pigment trait of over-riding importance in increasing the risk of cutaneous melanoma is the presence of proliferative melanocytic lesions, as indicated

Table 4. Risk of melanoma according to pigment cell phenotype, calculated from the conditional logistic model for matched pairs

Risk factor	β-Coefficient	Standard error	Relative risk	Confidence limits
Age	0.183			
Naevi, on arms	3.128	0.558	22.8	(7.6–68.1)
Lentigines on arms	1.000	0.437	2.7	(1.2– 6.4)
Propensity to sunburn	1.613	0.838	5.0	(1.0–25.9)
Little or no tan	0.643	0.498	1.9	(0.7– 5.0)
Hair colour (light brown/blonde)	1.340	0.565	3.8	(1.3–11.5)
Hair colour (red)	1.968	0.785	7.2	(1.5–33.3)
Eye colour (blue/grey)	0.173	0.456	1.2	(0.5– 2.9)
Eye colour (green/hazel)	0.257	0.478	1.3	(0.5– 3.3)
Fair skin colour (left forearm)	0.069	0.480	1.1	(0.4– 2.7)

here by observations on the arms. When the cutaneous phenotype is such that high-dose UVR is transmitted to a melanocyte prone to naevus formation in an individual also prone to sunburn without tanning, risks are exceptionally high – up to 51 times greater than when neither characteristic is present.

Familial and Genetic

Familial disposition to melanoma and presence of naevi and lentigines on the arms (probable phenotypic markers of atypical cell genotype) were assessed as genetic determinants of melanocyte proliferative tendencies. Familial predispositions to nonmelanoma skin cancers and to noncutaneous cancers were also assessed. Significantly more cases than controls had a positive family history of melanoma with a crude RR of 2.5 (1.3–4.7). There was no evidence of an association between melanoma and a positive family history of either skin cancer or cancer of other sites. There was little difference in risk according to the closeness of the familial relationship; having a first- or a second-degree relative with melanoma gave a similar RR. There was no association between melanoma and a positive family history after final adjustment using a logistic regression model; these findings are consistent with the hypothesis that risk of melanoma is associated with a family history which in turn is dependent on phenotypic and sun exposure factors (Green et al. 1985a). Thus, familial risk could be related to the propensity to common naevi in some persons and not necessarily to syndromes such as the dysplastic naevus syndrome (Elder et al. 1980). The assumption that naevi and lentigines indicate the genotype of the melanocyte may be limited by the extent to which their presence is determined by exposure to UVR. Risk factors for naevi and lentigines were therefore investigated in control subjects to explore the possible inter-relationships (Tables 5 and 6). Significant associations of naevi were: negatively with age; positively with propensity to freckle, large proportionate amounts of beach recreation at ages 10–19 years, and multiple sunburns in the whole of life. The association of lentigines with these factors, as well as with teenage sunburn experiences and actinic lesions on the face could be due in part to the difficulty in distinguishing between lentigines

Table 5. Associations between presence of naevi and lentigines on the arms and age. Phenotypic risk factors, ethnicity, and family history of melanoma in 183 control subjects

Risk factor level		Control subjects				
		Total	Proportion with naevi on arms		Proportion with lentigines on arms	
			No.	Percentage of total	No.	Percentage of total
Age (years)	<35	46	20	44	23	50
	35-49	58	12	21	17	29
	50+	79	14	18**	21	27*
Propensity to freckle	Absent	137	27	20	25	18
	Present	46	19	41**	36	78**
Depth of maximum tan	Dark	68	12	18	9	13
	Medium-light	104	31	30	46	44
	None	11	3	27	6	55**
Propensity to sunburn	Tan only	31	5	16	4	13
	Burn, tan	58	12	21	14	24
	Burn, peel	94	29	31	43	46**
Eye colour	Brown	52	15	29	12	23
	Green/hazel	47	13	28	20	43
	Blue/grey	82	18	22	29	35
Hair colour	Black/dark brown	47	11	23	13	28
	Light brown/blonde	121	28	23	37	31
	Red	15	7	47	11	73*
Skin colour on left forearm	Olive	48	9	19	6	13
	Fair	135	37	27	55	41*
Ethnicity of grandparents	Southern European	12	3	25	2	17
	Northern European	15	4	27	2	13
	United Kingdom	106	23	22	37	35
	Australian	50	16	32	20	40
Family history of melanoma	Absent	168	44	26	55	33
	Present	15	2	13	6	40

Significance of association [chi-square test or Bartholomew's test for trend (Bartholomew 1959)] as appropriate: *$P<0.05$; **$P<0.01$

and freckles. The latter are related to sun exposure but are not proliferative melanocytic lesions. Very high lifetime sun exposure was negatively associated with both lentigines and naevi on the arms. In part this is attributable to the negative association between naevi and age, but could also indicate that persons who have skin that is sensitive to the sun consciously avoid prolonged sun exposure as they grow older.

These positive findings among control subjects may indicate that naevi and lentigines are causally associated with other study factors. They provide some support for the concept that these lesions are part of the natural history of melanoma (Eng 1983; Holman et al. 1983). If this were so, then controlling for naevi and lentigines in an effort to take account of genotype in the analysis would reduce the calculated strength of association be-

Table 6. Associations between presence of naevi and lentigines on the arms and sun exposure factors in 183 control subjects

Sun exposure factor	Exposure level	Control subjects				
		Total	Proportion with naevi on arms		Proportion with lentigines	
			Number	Percentage of total	Number	Percentage of total
Proportionate beach	0-29%	131	23	18	34	26
recreation	30%-49%	7	4	57	4	57
10-19 years	50+%	45	19	42**	23	51**
Proportionate summer	0-29%	119	28	24	30	25
and beach recreation	30%-49%	27	6	22	12	44
Lifetime	50+%	37	12	32	19	50**
10-19 years	0%-29%	97	18	19	23	24
	30%-49%	9	3	33	6	67
	50+%	77	25	33	32	42**
5-years before case	0-29%	69	16	23	24	35
diagnosis	30%-49%	16	3	19	4	25
	50+%	98	27	28	33	34
Number of sunburn episodes	0-1	128	26	20	30	23
Lifetime	2-5	33	15	46	17	52
	6+	22	5	23	14	64**
10-19 years	0-1	139	30	22	35	25
	2-5	25	13	52	14	56
	6+	19	3	16	12	63**
Total sun exposure	<2000	21	10	48	13	62
Lifetime	2000-	130	30	23	42	32
	50000+	32	6	19*	6	19**
10-19 years	<500	52	14	27	24	46
	500-	81	23	28	29	36
	5000+	50	9	18	8	16**
5 years before case	<500	75	21	28	24	32
diagnosis	500-	91	20	22	30	33
	5000+	17	5	29	7	41
Actinic tumours on face	None	160	40	25	48	30
	Few	13	4	31	8	62
	Moderate/ many	7	1	14	5	71**

Significance of association [chi-square test or Bartholomew's test for trend (Bartholomew 1959)] as appropriate: $*P<0.05$; $**P<0.01$

tween UVR dosage and melanoma. The approach taken has been that naevi on the arms best represent inherent proliferative propensities of melanocytes. Lentigines on the arms appeared to be so strongly associated with, and indeed consequent upon, sun exposure that their inclusion in the model could have led to inappropriate reduction of the association between UVR and melanoma.

Sun Exposure

There was no association between melanoma and overall occupational sun exposure. In the spectrum of outdoor recreations generally available in Queensland, beach recreation is possibly unique, because of the high amounts of sun exposure involved. UVR reflectance of sand and sea results in very high levels of background radiation, the effects of which are heightened by the small amount of clothing worn. Table 7 shows the frequency distribution of hours spent on the beach in the sun during different life periods and the associated RRs, crude and adjusted, for the presence of naevi and age. No strong associations with melanoma were observed. There thus appears to be no important trend of increased risk associated with beach recreation considered in isolation during early, recent or total life periods. However, beach exposure needs to be placed in the context of other recreational and occupational sun exposure. The risks of cumulative hours of total sun exposure during different life periods are presented in Table 8. Stratified analysis performed on these grouped data showed no material confounding or modification of effect by age, sex or geographical location, gauged by the stratum-specific risk estimates. The final adjustment RR under the logistic model was 3.2 (0.9–12.4) for intermediate levels of sun exposure and 5.3 (0.9–30.8) for high sun exposure throughout life (Green 1984). There was a significant association with heavy sun exposure in the second decade; after stratified analysis adjusting for age and naevi on the arms, the RR was 4.4 (1.8–184.5). No association was seen with sun exposure in the 5 years prior to case diagnosis, however. When the joint effects of high total sun exposure and the presence of naevi of the arms were examined, trends of increasing risk with increasing sun exposure throughout life were seen, although point estimates of effect were greater when naevi were present.

Information on UVR levels in different places of residence was used to examine the total UVR exposure and its relationship to melanoma. However, there was no important modification of the relationship of cumulated sun hours for any period of life examined, suggesting that residential history was not markedly different in cases and controls.

Table 7. Recreational hours spent on the beach in the sun during different life periods and associated risk of melanoma, crude and adjusted for presence of naevi on the arms and age

Life period	Hours on beach	Cases	Controls	Relative Risk	
				Crude[a]	Adjusted
Whole of life	0	18	13	1.0	1.0
	1–	79	72	0.8	0.6[b] (0.2–1.4)[c]
	500–	70	92	0.5	0.3 (0.1–0.8)
	5000–	16	6	1.9	1.3[b] (0.4–4.3)
Ages 10–19 years	0	54	64	1.0	1.0
	1–	99	85	1.4	1.1 (0.6–2.0)
	500–	30	34	1.0	0.8[b] (0.4–1.9)
The 5 years prior to case diagnosis	0	61	49	1.0	1.0
	1–	104	122	0.7	0.6[b] (0.0–1.0)
	500–	18	12	1.2	0.9[b] (0.3–3.1)

[a] Relative risk calculated ignoring individual matching
[b] 0.5 added to each cell in stratum where any one cell contained zero
[c] 95% confidence limits

Table 8. Cumulative hours of sun exposure during different life periods and risk of melanoma

Life period	Cumulative sun hours	Cases	Controls	Relative risk	
				Crude[a]	Adjusted[c]
Whole of life	<2000	12	21	1.0	1.0
	2000–	78	78	1.7	2.3 (1.0–5.1)[d]
	50000–	31	24	2.3	1.7[b] (0.4–7.8)
Ages 10–19 years	<500	42	52	1.0	1.0
	500–	70	81	1.1	1.0 (0.5–2.0)
	5000–	41	21	1.8	4.4 (1.8–184.5)
The 5 years prior to case diagnosis	<500	87	74	1.0	1.0
	500–	78	92	0.7	0.9 (0.5–1.6)
	5000–	12	10	0.9	1.2[b] (0.5–2.9)

[a] Relative risk calculated ignoring individual matching
[b] 0.5 added to each cell of a stratum when any one cell contained zero
[c] Adjusted for age and presence of naevi on the arms
[d] 95% confidence limits

Chronic Sun Exposure

The presence of skin cancers and keratoses on the skin may be used as a direct measure of high chronic UVR dosage to the level of the melanocyte. A crude association was found between such "actinic tumours" and cutaneous melanoma, with an RR of 3.2 for the presence of actinic tumours on the forearm and 4.2 for their presence on the face. When age and presence of naevi on the arms were included in the logistic model, RR when actinic tumours were present on the face was 2.8 (1.1–7.2). There is not necessarily a direct correlation between exposure of the hands or face and that of melanocytes at the site of the particular melanomas. The data suggest that amongst persons who have experienced sun exposure over many years the resultant high UVR dosage is strongly associated with cutaneous melanoma (Green and O'Rourke 1985).

Sunburn

Severe sunburn is an indicator par excellence of acute excessive UVR dosage to the basal epidermis, similar to evidence of chronic high UVR dosage to this region provided by BCCs and SCCs. As the melanocyte is situated in the basal epidermis, these factors were used as direct indications that an excessive UVR dose had been received by the melanocyte despite any degree of filtering by the melanin in the overlying epidermis. A positive association between repeated sunburns and melanoma would support the hypothesis that intermittent intense exposure, i.e., high-dose rates of solar radiation to the target cells, is a significant factor in aetiology. In this study severe sunburn was defined as an episode in which pain had persisted for longer than 48 h with or without blistering. Up to nine sunburn experiences, together with the principal sites affected, were recorded for each decade of life.

In general, patients experienced more episodes of sunburn than controls. Multiple episodes of sunburn were commoner in cases than controls, with an RR of 1.5 (0.7–3.2) for

Table 9. Risk of melanoma at specific sites by multiple sunburn episodes at same or any site

Site of melanoma	Case-control pairs	Multiple sunburns	
		At site of melanoma	At any site
Head and neck	20[a]	3.0[b] (0.5–17.2)	4.5 (1.2–17.1)
Back and shoulder	62	3.2 (1.5–6.7)	2.9 (1.4– 6.1)
Upper limb	25	20.4[c] (2.2–188.5)	3.5 (0.9–13.0)
Lower limb	52	1.2 (0.4–3.0)	2.2 (1.0– 4.9)
Chest and abdomen	24	3.3 (0.3–31.4)	2.3 (0.7– 4.5)

[a] Numbers of case-control pairs grouped in each site stratum
[b] Relative risk calculated ignoring individual matching
[c] 0.5 added to each cell in a stratum when any one cell contained zero

an intermediate (2–5) number of burns and 2.4 (1.0–6.1) for many (6+) sunburn episodes throughout life. Except for the upper limb, RRs did not vary appreciably with respect to body site of the melanoma, whether or not the sites of sunburn were considered (Table 9). These findings suggest that the risk of melanoma is higher among persons who have experienced repeated severe sunburns and that this risk is more than doubled among those sunburnt six times or more (Green et al. 1985). This is the case regardless of the propensity to naevi on the arms. These findings are in accord with those in the United States of America and Scotland (MacKie and Aitchison 1982) and provide further support for the theory that repeated episodes of intense sun exposure are associated with the development of melanoma other than LMM. Moreover, the sunburn action spectrum lies in the UVR range of solar radiation, which supports the view that it is this component of sunlight which significantly damages melanocytes. There is no evidence, however, of a strong association between those anatomical sites which are repeatedly sunburnt and subsequent sites of melanoma (Table 9), as might be expected if a direct carcinogenic action of UVR light on melanocyte DNA were postulated. This may simple reflect the small numbers in the site-specific strata, but could also support an indirect carcinogenic effect from such exposure. The latter concept fits with experimental observations where changes in the melanocyte population are seen in shielded ears of UVR irradiated mice (Rosdahl 1979) and such effects may be mediated through immunological pathways (Fisher and Kripke 1982). Whatever the mechanism, the findings have implications especially for younger age groups up to early adulthood, as almost all (97%) reported sunburn occurring prior to the age of 40 years – indeed 93% of these had not experienced severe sunburn beyond age 30.

Migrants

Information about country of birth and age of arrival of immigrants was obtained, together with the countries of birth of parents and grandparents. A "Celtic score" from 0 to 4 was constructed from the number of parents or grandparents born in Ireland or Scotland. There is no association between Celticity as so defined and risk of melanoma in our data (Table 10). The crude RR for melanoma among all migrants compared with native-born Australians was 0.6 (0.3–1.1). In relation to age on arrival in Australia, crude RRs indicated a possible increased risk among migrants who had lived in Australia for 40 years or more (Table 11), although there were only ten subjects in this category. When factors relat-

Table 10. Distribution of 183 cases of melanoma and 183 controls according to birth of grandparents in Ireland or Scotland and associated risk of melanoma, crude and adjusted for presence of naevi on the arms and age

No. of grandparents born in Ireland or Scotland	Cases	Controls	Relative risk[a]	
			Crude	Adjusted
0	138	145	1.0	1.0
1–2	37	32	1.2	1.0 (0.5–2.1)
3–4	8	6	1.4	0.9 (0.3–2.9)

[a] Relative risk calculated ignoring individual matching

Table 11. Age on arrival and of 17 migrant cases and 28 controls according to duration of residence in Australia and associated crude risk of melanoma

Risk factor Age on arrival in Australia (years)	Cases	Controls	Relative risks[a]
0	166	155	1.0
1–9	5	7	0.7
10–19	3	8	0.3
20–29	5	11	0.4
30+	4	2	1.9
All ages	17	28	0.6
Duration of residence in Australia (years)			
1–19	6 (35%)	8 (29%)	1.0
20–39	5 (29%)	16 (57%)	0.4
40–59	3 (18%)	2 (7%)	2.0
60+	3 (18%)	2 (7%)	2.0

[a] Relative risk calculated ignoring individual matching

ing to cutaneous phenotype and sun exposure were simultaneously controlled in a conditional logistic analysis for matched pairs the RR associated with migration to Australia was 0.3 (0.1–1.4).

UVR Barriers and Filters

The hypothesis was put forward that various conditions affecting the skin's surface (topical factors) were related to cutaneous melanoma insofar as they enhanced or modified the effects of solar UVR on the basal epidermis. Three topical factors were considered: sweat, because of the potentially harmful effects of its chemical components; the removal of naturally occurring surface filters of UVR, such as hair, layers of dirt, and dead skin of the stratum corneum; and the use of sunscreen lotions.

Subjects were asked to classify themselves as average, heavy or light sweaters in relation to other people during everyday activities and were also asked how often they worked up a sweat while out in the sun. The propensity to sweat was identical among cases and controls, but cases reported being in the sun with sweat on the skin more often than did con-

Table 12. Washing with soap and risk of melanoma, crude and adjusted, for presence of naevi on the arms and lifetime sun exposure

Season	Frequency of washing	Cases	Controls	Crude RR[a]	Relative risk[a] adjusted	
					For naevi on arms	For total sun exposure
Summer	Once a day or less	88	110	1.0	1.0	1.0
	More than once a day	95	73	1.6	1.2 (0.7–2.0)	1.7 (1.1–2.6)
Winter	Once a day or less	157	155	1.0	1.0	
	More than once a day	26	28	0.9	0.9 (0.5–1.6)	

[a] Relative risk calculated ignoring individual matching

trols. The crude RR for melanoma associated with sweating in the sun two or more times per week was 1.8 (1.2–2.7). A multivariate analysis which included age, naevi, hair colour, propensity to sunburn, total sun exposure and propensity to sweat gave an RR for the last two of 2.0 (0.9–4.5).

There was little evidence to support an association between melanoma and the removal of natural filters of UVR radiation. In all cases hair was removed among women by shaving. Although the frequencies were generally the same in cases and controls when all sites were considered, an analysis restricted to the lower limbs showed a crude RR of 1.8 associated with regular leg shaving. However there was no increase in risk with an increased frequency of shaving and adjustment for naevi and for total sun exposure by stratified analysis made no appreciable difference. The use of multivariate analysis controlling jointly for several phenotypic and sun exposure factors reduced the RR for leg shaving on the lower limbs to 1.0 (0.2–5.7).

Washing with soap was investigated (Table 12) by asking about frequencies of bathing or showering with soap during the summer and winter as well as shampooing the hair under the shower. The last was asked to assess any possible irritant effects of detergent lather on melanocytes of the back and shoulders. Frequent washing in summer was associated with an increased risk of 1.6. Multivariate analysis including cutaneous phenotype and sun exposure produced an odds ratio of 1.3 in relation to washing (0.6–2.7). No association was observed between melanoma and washing during winter; neither was an association found with shampooing of the hair under a shower. Grouping all brands of UVR blocking agents together produced a crude RR of 1.0 and, after multivariate modelling with adjustment for UVR dosage and naevi, an RR of 0.8 (0.4–1.7).

The findings suggest that there may be a twofold increase in the risk of melanoma among those who are more often out in the sun with sweat on the skin when UVR dosage, naevi on the arms, and propensity to sweat are taken into account. Although the final estimates of risk were not statistically significant, this question merits further investigation. It is possible that sweating in the sun may be an indicator of intense or prolonged exposure to sunlight not measured in any other way; it is also possible, however, that sweat contains a carcinogenic photoproduct, and investigations of the composition of sweat after UVR

Table 13. Risk of melanoma by sex according to cigarette, coffee, tea and alcohol consumption

Risk factor	Exposure level	Crude RR[a]			Adjusted RR[b]
		Male	Female	Total	
Cigarette consumption	Rarely/never	1.0	1.0	1.0	1.0
	Ever	1.0	0.5	0.8	
Lifetime number of packs	1	0.5	0.7	0.6	0.7 (0.2–2.1)
	500–	0.6	1.1	0.8	0.8 (0.3–2.4)
	10000+	1.0	0.5	1.3	1.3 (0.3–5.0)
Coffee, cups/day	0			1.0	1.0
	1–4			0.9	0.9 (0.5–1.6)
	5+			1.0	
Tea, cups/day	0			1.0	1.0
	1–4			1.1	0.9 (0.4–1.6)
	5+			0.8	
Alcohol,	Rare/never	1.0	1.0	1.0	
units (15 ml absolute	Regular	0.6	1.1	0.9	
alcohol) month	1–	0.6	1.1	0.9	0.7 (0.2–1.7)
	50–	0.7	1.3	1.0	1.0 (0.3–3.2)
	100–	0.6	0.8	0.7	
	200+	0.6	0.3	0.7	0.6 (0.2–1.8)
Beer,	1–			0.9	
10 oz glasses/month	40–			0.9	
	80–			0.9	1.0 (0.7–1.4)
	200+			0.5	
Wine,	1–			0.7	
4 oz. glasses/month	40–			0.8	0.7 (0.4–1.2)
	80+			1.0	
Spirits,	1–			0.8	
1 oz. glasses/month	40			1.9	0.9 (0.5–1.6)
	80+			0.8	

[a] Relative risk calculated ignoring individual matching
[b] Relative risk calculated using matched data and adjusted for pigment cell phenotype and lifetime sun exposure

would be of interest. The effect of washing, with presumed removal of surface filters, was at most small.

The findings in relation to sun lotions suggest a possible protective effect when any kind of preparation is applied to the skin prior to sun exposure. However, these results were liable to substantial error because of the crude level of data obtained. Many more details regarding frequency, duration, and types of various agents used would be needed to obtain valid estimates of effect in relation to melanoma. The questions asked did not allow for the changes that have taken place over recent decades in the use of sun lotions, and future studies would need to take these into account to evaluate the overall effect of such agents.

Table 14. Risk of melanoma according to miscellaneous personal factors

Personal factor	Exposure level	Crude RR	Adjusted RR[a]
History of noncutaneous cancer	Absent	1.0	1.0
	Present	0.2	0.1 (0.0–1.7)
Age of diagnosis of other cancer (years)	30–39	0.1	
	40–59	0.6	
	60+	0.3	
Region of other cancer	Head/neck	0.2	
	Breast/lung	0.5	
	Kidney/bowel	0.2	
	Genital	0.2	
Excess weight (kg gain since age 21 years)	<3	1.0	1.0
	3–9	1.0	1.4 (0.6–3.7)
	10–19	1.0	1.4 (0.4–4.4)
	20+	1.3	1.4 (0.3–6.6)
Marital status	Never married	1.0	1.0
	Ever married	1.0	2.5 (0.7–8.2)[b]
	Married/de facto	1.0	
	Widowed	0.7	
Number of stressful life events in previous 5–6 years	0	1.0	1.0
	1–4	1.0	1.0 (1.0–2.2)[c]
	5–7	0.5	0.6 (0.1–4.9)
Use of permanent hair dyes (females)	Never	1.0	1.0
	Ever	0.8	0.9 (0.3–3.0)
Age at first use (years)	<20	2.5	
	20–39	0.4	
	40–59	0.5	

[a] Relative risk calculated ignoring individual matching
[b] Social class variable also included in the model
[c] Social class and marital status variables also included in the model

Hormones

Results of the analysis of the women's menstrual and child-bearing histories and hormonal therapy (Green and Bain 1985) showed no increased risk of melanoma in women associated with their ever having used OCs, and no significant positive associations were found when duration of OC use, age of last use or interval since use were considered. Further, no coherent positive relationship was found between melanoma and age at menarche, parity, or age at first birth when variables were considered separately or in the multivariate model controlling for phenotypic and sun exposure variables.

Miscellaneous Factors

Information on social and personal factors included marital status, cigarette, alcohol, tea and coffee consumption, and use of permanent hair dyes. The results are given in Tables 13 and 14. There was no increased risk of melanoma apparent among cigarette smokers in general or when they were graded by lifetime cigarette consumption. The distribution of daily intake of tea and coffee was virtually the same among cases and controls; adjusting for naevi and UVR dosage made little difference to this finding. Similarly, there was no evidence of increased risk associated with alcohol consumed regularly or with specific types of beverages (beer, wine or spirits). A history of noncutaneous cancer had an age-adjusted RR of 0.1. There was little different in marital status between cases and controls, although adjustment for UVR dosage and naevi resulted in a nonsignificant RR of 2.5 for the ever married. There was some increase in estimates of RR with weight-gain since age 21. The use of hair dyes in women showed no association with melanoma. There was also a lower risk among those with a large number of stressful life events, but this was not statistically significant.

These findings do not suggest that any of a range of social and personal factors are important risk factors for melanoma. High social status as indicated by occupation and level of education was not associated with increased risk as reported by others (Holman et al. 1980; Lee and Strickland 1980).

Information was collected on X-irradiation other than diagnostic X-rays, on medication, and on exposure to chemicals in the environment. There was no evidence of an association between therapeutic radiation and melanoma. Prescribed drugs were not associated with melanoma, although risk estimates could not be given due to small numbers. There was no increased risk for general exposure to environmental chemicals, but again the numbers were too small for analysis of specific exposures.

Conclusion

Evidence is presented that a marker of significant risk for melanoma is the presence of common acquired naevi on the arms. Other characteristics of pigment phenotype are confirmed as risk factors for melanoma. Observations that subjects with pale and sun-sensitive complexions, signified by light hair colour and a propensity to sunburn on acute exposure, are more likely to develop melanoma offer support for the solar UVR hypothesis regarding aetiology. Furthermore, it was found that solar UVR in a large dosage accumulated over a lifetime is associated with the development of melanoma. The high UVR dosage may be the result of heavy sun exposure over the long term, or repeated episodes of severe short-term exposures. It is also possible that, after UVR exposure, sweat contains a carcinogen which has a causal role in melanoma development. Exposure to miscellaneous environmental chemicals may be important as well. Occupational status, cigarette and alcohol consumption, and hormonal exposures do not appear to be significant determinants of risk, after the major phenotypic and environmental factors are taken into account.

References

Acquavella JF, Pietjen GL, Wilkinson GS (1982) Malignant melanoma incidence at the Los Alamos National Laboratory. Lancet 1: 883-884

Adam SA, Sheaves JK, Wright NH et al. (1981) A case-control study of the possible association between oral contraceptives and malignant melanoma. Br J Cancer 44: 45-50

Ariel IM (1980) Theories regarding the cause of malignant melanoma. Surg Gynecol Obstet 150: 907-917

Armstrong BK, McNulty JC, Levitt LJ et al. (1979) Mortality in gold and coal miners in Western Australia with special reference to lung cancer. Br J Ind Med 36: 199-205

Armstrong BK, Holman CDJ, Ford JM, Woodings TL (1982) Trends in melanoma incidence and mortality in Australia. In: Magnus K (ed) Trends in cancer incidence: causes and practical implications. Hemisphere, New York, pp 399-417
Ashwood-Smith MJ, Poulton GA, Barker M, Mildenberger M (1980) 5-Methoxypsoralen, an ingredient in several suntan preparations, has lethal, mutagenic and clastogenic properties. Nature 285-407-409
Austin DF, Reynolds PJ, Snyder MA et al. (1981) Malignant melanoma among employees of Lawrence Livermore National Laboratory. Lancet 2: 712-716
Bahn AK, Rosenwaike I, Hermann N, et al. (1976) Melanoma after exposure to PCB's. N Engl J Med 295-450
Bain C, Hennekens C, Speizer FC et al. (1982) Oral contraceptive use and malignant melanoma. JNCI 68: 537-539
Bartholomew DJ (1959) A test of homogeneity for ordered alternatives. Biometrika 46: 36-48
Barton IJ, Paltridge GW (1979) The Australian climatology of biologically effective ultraviolet radiation. Aust J Dermatol 55: 85-87
Beardmore GL (1982) Keratoses. In: Emmett AJ, O'Rourke MG (eds) Malignant skin tumours. Churchill Livingstone. Edinburgh, pp 95-101
Beral V, Ramcharan S, Faris R (1977) Malignant melanoma and oral contraceptive use among women in California. Br J Cancer 36: 804-809
Beral V, Evans S, Shaw H, Milton G (1982) Malignant melanoma and exposure to fluorescent lighting at work. Lancet 2: 290-293
Birkmayer GD, Balda BR, Miller F (1974) Oncorna viral information in human melanoma. Eur J Cancer 10: 419-424
Black HS, Douglas DR (1972) A model system for the evaluation of the role of cholesterol α-oxide in ultraviolet carcinogenesis. Cancer Res 32: 2630-2632
Black HS, Lo WB (1971) Formation of a carcinogen in human skin irradiated in ultraviolet light. Nature 234: 306-308
Bork K, Brauninger W, Nake A (1981) Increased frequency of multiple primary melanomas in hereditary familial melanoma. Dermatologia 162: 191-196
Breslow NE, Day NE (1980) Statistical methods in cancer research, vol 1: the analysis of case-control studies. IARC Sci Publ 32: 248-279
Chan J, Black HS (1976) Distribution of cholesterol-5a, 6a-epoxide formation and its metabolism in mouse skin. J Invest Dermatol 66: 112-116
Chaudhuri PK, Walker MJ, Briele HA, Beatti OW, Das Gupta TK (1980) Incidence of oestrogen receptors in benign nevi and human malignant melanoma. JAMA 244: 791-793
Clark WH, Mastrangelo MJ, Ainsworth AM, Berd D, Bellet RE, Bernardino EA (1977) Current concepts of the biology of human cutaneous malignant melanoma. Adv Cancer Res 24: 267-338
Clough P (1980) Incidence of malignant melanoma of the skin in England and Wales. Br Med J 2: 112
Cornfield J (1951) A method of estimating comparative rates from clinical data: applications to cancer of the lung, breast and cervix. JNCI 11: 1269-1275
Daniels F (1969) Optics of the skin as related to ultraviolet radiation. In: Urbach F (ed) The biologic effects of ultraviolet radiation. Pergamon, Oxford, pp 151-157
Dubreuilh MW (1912) De la mélanose circonscrite précancereuse. Ann Dermatol Syph (Paris) 3: 129
Elwood JM, Lee JAH (1979) Recent data on the epidemiology of malignant melanoma. In: Clark W, Goldman L, Mastrengelo M (eds) Human malignant melanoma. Grune and Stratton, New York, pp 261-272
Elder DE, Goldman LI, Goldman SC et al. (1980) Dysplastic nevus syndrome: a phenotypic association of sporadic cutaneous melanoma. Cancer 46: 1787-1794
Elder DE, Kraemer KH, Greene MH, Clark WH, Guerry D (1982) The dysplastic nevus syndrome: our definition. Am J Dermatopathol 4: 455-460
Eng AM (1983) Solitary small active junctional naevi in juvenile patients. Arch Dermatol 119: 35-38
Farber E (1981) Chemical carcinogenesis. N Engl J Med 305: 1379-1389

Feibleman CE, Stoll H, Maize JC (1980) Melanomas of the palm, sole, and nail bed: a clinicopathologic study. Cancer 46: 2492-2504

Fisher MS, Kripke ML (1982) Suppressor T-lymphocytes control the development of primary skin cancers in ultraviolet irradiated mice. Science 216: 1133-1134

Forbes P, Davis R, Urbach F (1979) Aging, environmental influences and photocarcinogenesis. J Invest Dermatol 73: 131-134

Gilchrest BA, Blog FB, Szabo G (1979) Effects of aging and chronic sun exposure on melanocytes in human skin. J Invest Dermatol 73: 141-143

Green A (1984) Sun exposure and the risk of melanoma. Aust J Dermatol 25: 99-102

Green A, Bain C (1985) Hormonal factors and melanoma in women. Med J Aust 142: 446-448

Green A, O'Rourke M (1985) Cutaneous malignant melanoma in association with other skin cancers. JNCI 74: 977-980

Green A, Siskind V (1983) Geographical distribution of cutaneous melanoma in Queensland. Med J Aust 1: 407-410

Green A, MacLennan R, Siskind V (1985 a) Common acquired naevi and the risk of malignant melanoma. Int J Cancer 35: 297-300

Green A, Siskind V, Bain C, Alexander J (1985 b) sunburn and malignant melanoma. Br J Cancer 51: 393-397

Happle R, Traupe H, Vakilzadeh F, Macher E (1982) Polygenic inheritance and precursor nevi. J Am Acad Dermatol 6: 540-543

Helmrich SP, Rosenberg L, Kaufman DW (1984) Lack of elevated risk of malignant melanoma in relation to oral contraceptive use. JNCI 72: 617-620

Hoar SK, Pell S (1981) A retrospective cohort study of mortality and cancer incidence among chemists. J Occup Med 23: 485-495

Holly EA, Weiss NS, Liff J (1983) Cutaneous malignant melanoma in relation to exogenous hormones and reproductive factors. JNCI 70: 827-831

Holman CDJ, James IR, Gattey PH et al. (1980) An analysis of trends in mortality from malignant melanoma of the skin in Australia. Int J Cancer 26: 703-709

Holman CDJ, Heenan PJ, Caruso V, Glancy RJ, Armstrong BK (1983) Seasonal variation in the junctional component of pigmented naevi. Int J Cancer 31: 213-215

Horrobin DF, Troska JE (1981) The possible effect of diazepam on cancer development and growth. Med Hypotheses 7: 115-125

Jimbow K, Uesugi T (1982) New melanogenesis and photobiological processes in activation and proliferation of precursor melanocytes after UV exposure. J Invest Dermatol 78: 108-115

Lee JAH (1982) Melanoma and exposure to sunlight. Epidemiol Rev 4: 110-136

Lee JAH, Storer BE (1980) Excess of malignant melanomas in women in the British Isles. Lancet 2: 1337-1339

Lee JAH, Strickland D (1980) Malignant melanoma: social status and outdoor work. Br J Cancer 41: 757-763

Little JH, Holt J, Davis N (1980) Changing epidemiology of malignant melanoma in Queensland. Med J Aust 1: 66-69

Mantel N, Haenszel W (1959) Statistical aspects of the analysis of data from retrospective studies of disease. JNCI 22: 719-748

MacKie RM, Aitchison T (1982) Severe sunburn and subsequent risk of primary cutaneous melanoma in Scotland. Br J Cancer 46: 955-960

McCarthy WH (1981) Excessive washing and melanoma. Med J Aust 1: 716

McGovern VJ (1977) Epidemiological aspects of melanoma: a review. Pathology 9: 233-241

McGovern VJ, Shaw HM, Milton GW, Farago GA (1980) Is malignant melanoma arising in a Hutchinson's melanotic freckle a separate disease entity? Histopathology 4: 235-242

McNeer G, Das Gupta TK (1964) Prognosis in malignant melanoma. Surgery 56: 512-518

Miller TR, Pack GT (1962) The familial aspect of malignant melanoma. Arch Dermatol 86: 35-39

Mitchell R (1963) The effect of prolonged solar radiation on melanocytes of the human epidermis. J Invest Dermatol 41: 199-212

Neifield JP, Lippman ME (1980) Steroid receptors and malignant melanoma. J Invest Dermatol 74: 379-381

Paltridge GW, Barton IJ (1978) Erythemal ultraviolet radiation distribution over Australia - the calculation, detailed results and input frequency analysis of observed Australian cloud cover. CSIRO Aust Div Phys Tech Pap 33, Melbourne

Parsons PG, Klucis E, Goss PD, Pope JH, Little JH, Davis NC (1976) Oncornavirus-like particles in malignant melanoma and control biopsies. Int J Cancer 18: 757-763

Pinkus H (1971) Epithelial neoplasms and precancerous lesions. In: Fitzpatrick TB, Arndt KA, Clark WH, Eisen AZ, Van Scott EJ, Vaughan JS (eds) Dermatology in general medicine. McGraw-Hill, New York, pp 399-407

Pinkus H (1976) Anatomy and embryology of the skin. In: Andrade R, Gumport S, Papkin G, Rees T (eds) Cancer of the skin. Saunders, Philadelphia, pp 16-83

Quevedo WC, Szabo G, Virks J, Sinesi SJ (1965) Melanocyte populations in UV-irradiated human skin. J Invest Dermatol 45: 295-298

Ramsay R, Chen P, Imray P, Kidson C, Lavin M, Hockey A (1982) Familial melanoma associated with dominant ultraviolet radiation sensitivity. Cancer Res 42: 2909-2912

Reynolds P, Austin D, Thomas J (1982) Familial and occupational risks of malignant melanoma (Abs). Am J Epidemiol 116: 570

Rosdahl IK (1979) Local and systemic effects on the epidermal melanocyte population in UV-irradiated mouse skin. J Invest Dermatol 73: 306-309

Rosdahl IK, Szabo G (1978) Mitotic activity of epidermal melanocytes in UV-irradiated mouse skin. J Invest Dermatol 70: 143-148

Schulze R (1978) Measurement of sunlight: the ultraviolet B radiation in sunlight. In: Kripke ML, Sass ER (eds) International conference on ultraviolet carcinogenesis. National Institutes of Health, Bethesda, p 214 (NIH publication no 78-1532)

Shiu MH, Schottenfeld D, Maclean B, et al. (1976) Adverse effect of pregnancy on melanoma. Cancer 37: 181-187

Snell RS (1967) Hormonal control of pigmentation in man and other mammals. In: Montagna W, Hu F (eds) The pigmentary system. Pergamon, New York (Advances in biology of the skin, vol VIII)

Szabo G (1967) The regional anatomy of the human integument with special reference to the distribution of hair follicles, sweat glands, and melanocytes. Phil Trans R Soc Lond 282B: 447

Thomas TL, Decoufle P (1979) Mortality among workers employed in the pharmaceutical industry: a preliminary investigation. J Occup Med 21: 619-623

White LP (1959) Studies on melanoma II: sex and survival in human melanoma. N Engl J Med 260: 789-797

Williams RR (1976) Breast and thyroid cancer and malignant melanoma promoted by alcohol-induced pituitary secretion of prolactin, TSH and MSH. Lancet 1: 996-999

Zajdela F, Bisagni E (1981) 5-Methoxypsoralen, the melanogenic additive in sun-tan preparations is tumorigenic in mice exposed to 365 nm U.V. radiation. Carcinogenesis 2: 121-127

Occupation and Malignant Melanoma of the Skin*

D. F. Austin and P. Reynolds

Cancer Prevention Section, California State Department of Health Services, 5850 Shellmound Street, Suite 200, Emeryville, CA 94608, USA

Introduction

Occupational risks for malignant melanoma (MM) of the skin have not been systematically studied. Epidemiologic research on MM has focused on sunlight exposure, even though available evidence shows that, unlike most other cancers in general and other cancers of the skin in particular, MM tends to be associated with indoor work, upper socioeconomic status, and particularly technical-professional occupations (Beral and Robinson 1981; Lee and Strickland 1980; Teppo et al. 1980). These findings have been largely dismissed by appealing to postulated differences in leisure-time sun exposure in these occupational groups. New evidence suggests, however, that the occupational epidemiology of MM is an area in serious need of further study.

MM is a cancer which has been rapidly increasing, especially among men in the San Francisco Bay area, and in the last several years we have experienced several instances of what appear to be MM "clusters" in occupational groups (Austin et al. 1981; Austin 1982). The most publicized of these was the excess among employees of the Lawrence Livermore National Laboratory (LLNL), which prompted us to reevaluate the available information on occupational associations with MM and its concordance with findings from our study of MM among LLNL employees (Austin and Reynolds 1984). To our knowledge, the LLNL study is the first occupational study of MM which attempts to assess occupational contributions to MM risk while controlling for constitutional and life-style factors.

We have reviewed a variety of studies for information on potential occupational risks for MM. These include: (a) ecologic studies; (b) standardized or proportional mortality and proportional incidence studies of cancer drawn from registry or vital data; (c) cohort mortality studies; (d) cohort incidence studies; and (e) case-control studies of MM.

Ecologic Studies

A number of studies have examined geographic patterns of sunlight exposure and MM incidence, but few have examined industry-associated clustering. Two rather well-known studies of cancer-industry associations (Blot et al. 1977; Hoover and Fraumeni 1975) are summarized with regard to their MM findings in Table 1.

* *Abbreviations: PMR,* proportionate mortality ratio; *SMR,* standardized mortality ratio; *OR,* odds ratio; *MM,* malignant melanoma

Recent Results in Cancer Research. Vol 102

Table 1. Ecologic associations with malignant melanoma of the skin

Year	Author	Outcome	Association
1975	Hoover and Fraumeni 1975	Mortality	10% elevation of MM among males and females in counties with *chemical industries* ($P<0.05$)
1977	Blot et al. 1977	Mortality	MM + other skin cancer, ratio of age-adjusted mortality rates in white males = 1.10 ($P<0.05$) in counties with *petrochemical industries*

In their 1975 study of cancer mortality rates in U.S. counties with chemical industries, Hoover and Fraumeni (1975) noted a significant elevation of MM deaths in these counties. In a similarly designed later study, Blot et al. (1977) noted a significantly elevated ratio of general skin cancer mortality among men living in certain counties with petrochemical industries compared with "control" counties (demographically similar but without petrochemical industry).

Standardized or Proportional Incidence and Mortality Studies

Table 2 summarizes the general evidence from a number of studies exploring the occupational distribution within cancer incidence or mortality series (Adelstein 1972; Austin and Reynolds, in preparation; CCER 1980; Decoufle and Stanislawczyk 1977; Dubrow and Wegman, 1984; Logan 1982; Mack, T., personal communication; Milham 1976; Peterson and Milham 1980; Stellman and Garfinkel 1984; Williams et al. 1977).

Among the best known of these studies are those summarizing the decennial supplements on occupation and mortality which have been published by the Registrar General for Great Britain and Wales (Adelstein 1972; Logan 1982). Data in these reports have been presented as standardized mortality ratios (SMRs), proportiontionate mortality ratios (PMRs), and proportionate standardized mortality ratios (PSMRs). What is most striking for malignant melanoma mortality is the consistency, through time and with different risk measurements, of the gradient of risk by social class, with the highest risk in social class I ("professional" occupations), and the lowest risk in social class V (nonskilled manual labor). Equally striking is the contrast with the risk profile for nonmelanoma skin cancers, suggesting etiologic differences.

A similar effort in the United States is available in Milham's (1976) analysis of occupational mortality data for the state of Washington, replicated by Petersen and Milham (1980) in California. The Milham and Peterson analyses provide much more detailed information on specific occupational groups. Both present PMRs for white males. Some of the specific groups at highest risk include clergy, schoolteachers, clerical and kindred, a variety of white-collar groups, and carpenters. At significantly lower risk are laborers (Milham's PMR = 37). A similar analysis of the mortality experience for the state of Massachusetts by Dubrow and Wegman (1984) highlighted MM risk in the clergy, clerical and kindred workers, sales clerks, and especially among teachers, professors, school administrators, and other school professions.

Somewhat different in design is the American Cancer Society's (ACS) volunteer study. Although no general results on the mortality experience by occupation have been pub-

Table 2. Occupations associated with malignant melanoma cancer incidence and mortality surveys

Occupation	Mortality studies					Incidence studies				
	1	2	3	4	5	6	7	8	9	10
Administrators	++	+		+			+		+	+
Accountants		+	++						+	+
Clerical	++	+		+		+	+			
Paper/printing	++	+					+	+		
Teachers		++	+	+		++	+		+	++
Professors		+	+	+						++
Clergy		+		+			+		+	
Physicians/ dentists		+					+		+	
Lawyers/judges			+						+	+
Engineers		+	+				+			
Professional/ technical NOS	++					+	+			++
Armed forces	+	+					+	+		
Carpenters	+	++	+		+					

1, Adelstein (1972) and Logan (1982) UK; *2,* Milham (1976), Washington State; *3,* Peterson and Milham (1980) California; *4,* Dubrow and Wegman (to be published), Massachusetts; *5,* Stellman and Garfinkel (1984), American Cancer Society; *6,* Williams et al. (1977), Third National Cancer Survey; *7,* Committee for the Cancer-Environment, Sweden (1980); *8,* Decoufle and Stanislawczyk (1977) Roswell Park; *9,* Mack T., personal communication, Los Angeles County; *10,* Austin and Reynolds (to be published), San Francisco Bay area

lished, Stellman and Garfinkel's (1984) suggestive findings of enhanced MM risk among carpenters and joiners (SMR = 161) is consistent with the findings of Milham and Petersen.

A number of analyses have also been conducted of the occupational distribution in cancer incidence series. Williams et al. (1977) evaluated the relative distributions of industry and occupation among interviewed respondents drawn from a 10% sample of the Third National Cancer Survey (TNCS). Industries with significantly increased MM risk included communications and utilities (male OR = 11.3) and schools (female OR = 5.75; $P < 0.01$). The TNCS sample occupational data also underscore enhanced MM risk in professional-technical occupations, and especially the MM risk among female schoolteachers (OR = 5.06, $P < 0.05$).

Another source of special survey information comes from the analyses by Decoufle and Stanislawczyk (1977) of occupational associations by cancer site for a large series of Roswell Park cancer patients. Their findings suggest increased MM risks in the paper and printing industries and in the armed forces. While these findings are consistent with the mortality findings of Milham for Washington state and of Adelstein and Logan for the United Kingdom, the fact that this is the only such study failing to reveal, an observed association with professional-technical occupations may be due to the particular referral patterns of the case series.

Three population-based cancer registries have conducted proportional incidence ratio (PIR) analyses of occupational risks for different sites of cancer. These include the Swedish Cancer Registry (1980), the Los Angeles (California) Cancer Surveillance Program (Mack, T., personal communication), and the Surveillance, Epidemiology and End Results (SEER) Program in California (Austin and Reynolds, in preparation). The Swedish registry occupational data was obtained via record linkage between the cancer registry and census data. They reported increased MM risks similar to those from the Roswell Park series, in the paper and printing industry, and among members of the armed forces. In another analysis of the Swedish registry data white-collar workers were found to have significantly higher MM risks and blue-collar workers, significantly lower MM risks (Vagero and Persson 1984). The Los Angeles program routinely collects occupational information for newly diagnosed resident cancer cases. They have occupational information for 79% of white male and 43% of white female cases, and industry information for 67% of white male and 40% of white female cases. Among the most striking associations by industry are elementary and secondary schools (age-adjusted male PIR = 170, female PIR = 120), and legal services (male PIR = 210). Particular occupations at enhanced risk include lawyers (male PIR = 170), physicians (male PIR = 170, female PIR = 150), school administrators (male PIR = 350, female PIR = 150), chemists (male PIR = 270), and clergy and religious workers (male PIR = 210, female PIR = 290).

These general associations may also be consistent with a specific finding from the Atlanta Cancer Surveillance Program (Greenberg, R. personal communication). Greenberg noted a strikingly disproportionate number of health care workers among female MM cases diagnosed between 1975 and 1979. The PIR, compared with working women in the Atlanta SMSA, was 1.71 ($P = 0.01$). Notably, roughly one-quarter of these patients (5 of 21) were women in laboratory environments.

San Francisco-Oakland cancer registry data have been analyzed for age-adjusted PIRs for MM by industrial groups (Austin and Reynolds, in preparation). Although classification was by industry rather than occupation, the results are consistent with those from other population-based series. The greatest excesses are for professional-technical groups, particularly in educational institutions.

The evidence available from these mortality and incidence series varies widely with respect to time periods, sampling methods, ratio measurement procedures, occupational groupings, and occupational ascertainment methods. Given all these inconsistencies, coupled with the fact that the number of MM cases or deaths is reasonably small in each, the patterns of risk are remarkably consistent.

Cohort Mortality Studies

In studies conducted to evaluate cancer mortality in identified occupational cohorts, MM is seldom individually identified. However, some studies address skin cancer mortality (to which MM is frequently a major contributor) and a few recent studies include information on MM deaths.

Table 3 summarizes cohort studies with mention of skin cancer mortality (Hadjimichael et al. 1983; Matanoski et al. 1975; Thomas et al. 1980; Waxweiler et al. 1983). While these suggest that enhanced skin cancer risks may be possible, only one (Thomas et al. 1980) demonstrates a significant excess (in a petrochemical cohort).

In Table 4, cohort studies specifically reporting MM mortality are summarized (Armstrong et al. 1979; Caldwell et al. 1983; Greene et al. 1979; Olin et al. 1985; Rushton and Alderson 1981; Thomas and Decoufle 1979). Although only a small number of MM deaths are reported in each, some statistically significant MM excesses are reported across a variety of industrial cohorts, most notably in cohorts with probable risks for unusual chemical exposures.

Table 3. Occupational cohorts with excesses of skin cancer (including melanoma)

Year	Authors	Cohort	Outcome	O/E	Specific findings/ comments
1975	Matanoski et al.	Physicians	Mortality	-	Radiologists at excess risk for skin cancer, especially earlier cohorts
1980	Thomas et al.	OCAW Petrochemical workers (Texas)	Mortality	1.8*	Excess greater among members <10 years
1983	Waxweiler et al.	Petrochemical plant employees (Connecticut)	Mortality	1.1	Data for hourly, not salaried employees
1983	Hadjimichael et al.	Nuclear Fuels Fabricating (Connecticut)	Mortality Incidence	2.4 1.5	Excess evident for both industrial and office employees

* $P < 0.05$

Table 4. Occupational cohorts with excesses of malignant melanoma: mortality studies

Year	Authors	Cohort	MM deaths	O/E	Specific findings/ comments
1979	Armstrong et al.	Coal miners (Australia)	3	15.8*	Compared with male mortality in W. Australia
1979	Thomas and Deconfle	Pharmaceutical	6	3.5*	Excesses observed for males in production and administrative positions/no deaths among maintenance and engineering workers
1979	Greene et al.	Printing plant workers	4	1.5	Authors note presence of a number of possible exposures, including PCBs in ink
1981	Rushton and Alderson	Petrochemical workers (Great Britain)	14	2.2*	Compared with total mortality for England and Wales. Most of the MM deaths occurred at two of the eight study refineries with most among operators.
1983	Caldwell et al.	Nuclear test participants	2	5.0	Troops present at "Smoky" in 1957
1985	Olin et al.	Electrical engineers	3	3.2	Compared with a cohort of architects

* $P < 0.01$

Cohort Incidence Studies

Most of the cohort studies of cancer incidence which include information on MM are very recent and some are not yet published. These are summarized in Table 5 (Austin 1981; Bahn et al. 1976; Heldaas et al. 1984; Hilt et al. to be published; Hoar and Pell 1981; Holmberg et al. 1983; Pell et al. 1978; Vagero and Olin 1983; Vagero et al. 1985).

Table 5. Occupational cohorts with excesses of malignant melanoma: Incidence studies

Year	Authors	Cohort	Cases	O/E	Specific findings/ comments
1976	Bahn et al.	Petrochemical ("Northeast")	3	5.0**	Significant excess among men heavily exposed to PCBs; smaller excess among lightly exposed
1978	Pell et al.	DuPont employees	118	(Males) 1.2*	Excess same for wage and salary-earning males
			18	(Females) 1.2	Excess highest for salaried women
1981	Austin et al.	LLNL employees	17	(Males) 3.0*	Especially chemists
			2	(Females) 1.5	
1981	Hoar and Pell	DuPont chemists	8	2.4*	Significant excess compared with TNCS, nonsignificant compared with total nonchemist DuPont
1983	Holmberg et al.	Rubber Industry	21	2.3**	Excess is primarily among production workers not in weighing/mixing. White-collar O/E is elevated but not significantly so
1983	Vagero and Olin	Electronics Industry	59	1.4*	Excess in men only, compared with general working population
1984	Heldaas et al	Vinyl chloride and polyvinyl chloride workers	4	5.1*	Excess high in "high-exposure" group (O/E = 9.1)
1984	Hilt et al. (to be published)	Electrochemical plant (Nitric acid production workers)	3	5.1*	Overall excess, not confined to high asbestos exposure group (study group)
1985	Vagero et al.	Telecommunications Industry	12	2.6*	Especially with exposure to soldering

* $P < 0.05$; ** $P < 0.01$

Again, the number of MM cases observed in these occupational cohorts are generally small, the largest number coming from the DuPont Company's ongoing cancer registry program for active employees. Covering the time 1956-1974, these data are based on standardized incidence ratios (SIRs) computed for nearly 2 million person-years of observation (approximately 85% male). The reasonably large number of cases reported by Vagero (1983) were drawn from record linkage of the 1960 census of the population in Sweden to the Swedish Cancer Registry (cases for 1961-1973) to identify cases among workers in the electronic or electrical manufacturing industry. Similarly, all these studies except for that by Bahn et al. (1976) and the DuPont studies (Hoar and Pell 1981; Pell et al. 1978) are based on cohort record linkage to population-based cancer registry files. Our study (Austin et al. 1981) was based on record linkage between the Lawrence Livermore National Laboratory (LLNL, a high-energy physics research facility) and the SEER registry for the San Francisco-Oakland Metropolitan Statistical Area. The studies by Vagero's group (Vagero and Olin 1983; Vagero et al. 1985) and Holmberg (1983) were based on record linkage to the Swedish Cancer Registry, and the studies by Heldaas (1984) and Hilt (to be published) were based on record linkage to the Norwegian Tumor Registry.

With the exception of our study (Austin et al. 1981), none of these studies was designed as an a priori test for an excess of MM, but rather to evaluate patterns of general cancer risk. The most striking consistency across these studies is that significantly enhanced MM risks are in evidence in modern, technologically sophisticated occupational groups that are particularly characterized by a variety of chemical (and radiation) exposure risks not common in the general population.

Table 6. Case-control studies of malignant melanoma

Year	Authors	Study description	Odds ratio	Specific findings/ comments
1982	Elashoff et al.	Los Angeles and SF Bay area women, 15-55 years. Friend and neighbor controls. Unpublished results	1.2	Teachers
			4.8**	Operatives, laborers, farmers
			5.2*	Life and physical scientists
1983	Wright et al.	Chemists with MM vs chemists with other cancers, Los Angles	>27.0*	Benzoyl peroxide
			>13.5	Plastics, pesticides
			12.0*	Ionizing radiation
			7.5	Solvents
1983	Holman	W. Australia, 511 population-based case-control pairs, unpublished results		Occupational exposure to ionizing radiation
			2.7*	HMF melanoma (males)
			1.0	Superficial spreading melanoma (males)
1984	Green	Queensland, matched pairs, unpublished results	1.7*	Crude risk for chemical exposure, occupational
1984	Austin	LLNL workplace cluster investigation, unpublished results	9.4	Chemist duties
			4.5	Pacific Test Site
			3.6*	Volatile photochemicals
			3.4*	Radioactive materials
			1.8	"Site 300"

* $P<0.05$; ** $P<0.01$

Case-Control Studies

Few case-control studies of MM have explored specific occupational risk factors. Table 6 summarizes the evidence from five (Austin and Reynolds 1984; Elashoff et al. 1982; Green, A., unpublished data; Holman 1982; Wright et al. 1983) very recent case-control studies, for only one of which the occupational information is published (Wright et al. 1983).

The study by Elashoff (1982) was originally designed to test the association between oral contraceptive usage and MM, and the Holman (1982) and Green (unpublished data) studies were dissertation projects designed to explore general etiologic risks. These studies represent large case series, but the occupational information is minimal. The Wright (1983) and Austin (1984) studies were both designed to explore specific occupational exposures further in cohorts previously identified to be at excess risk. They are both characterized, however, by very small numbers: 9 case and 24 control chemists (chemists with other cancers) in the Wright study (1983) and 31 MM cases and 110 controls (LLNL employees, age/race/sex matched to the cases) in the Austin and Reynolds study (1984). Despite these limitations, together these studies suggest that occupational risks associated with similar chemical exposures or ionizing radiation may be important. The data from Holman's (1982) study suggest that these risks may be particularly relevant for lentigo maligna melanoma, or at least operate differently for different histologic types.

In our case-control study (Austin and Reynolds 1984) we attempted to evaluate the occupational contribution to MM risk independently of other known or suspected risk factors. The estimated odds ratios (estimated via conditional logistic regression) for each of the five occupational risk factors among LLNL employees were adjusted for the primary nonoccupational risk factors in this study group. As the risk coefficients associated with these five factors do not change appreciably with adjustment for constitutional risk or for each other, we assume they each make an independent occupational contribution to risk. Furthermore, there is evidence that these risk factors together may account for the approximate fourfold excess risk observed in this occupational cohort (Table 7).

Table 7. Predicted MM excess among LLNL employees, based on the magnitude of each putative causal occupational risk factor and its prevalence among LLNL employees

Factor	LLNL prevalence[a]	Relative risk[b]	Effect on LLNL rate[c]	Combined effect[d]
Radioactive materials	32.7%	3.38	178%	178%
Volatile photochemicals	15.5%	3.59	140%	249%
"Site 300" (weapons testing")	31.8%	1.75	124%	309%
Chemist duties	1.8%	9.37	115%	335%
Nuclear testing in the Pacific	3.6%	4.51	113%	400%

[a] Prevalence is that in the study controls

[b] Relative risk is the odds ratio, adjusted for matching and for all five other variables in the multivariate model

[c] Assuming that the prevalence of these risk factors in the general (non-LLNL) population is negligible: Relative rate = (LLNL prevalence) (RR) + (1-LLNL prevalence)

[d] Because the estimate of relative risk is derived from logistic regression the putative combined effects are multiplicative

Conclusions

Occupation has not previously been considered to be a major risk factor for MM, except as an indicator of socioeconomic status. Insofar as MM has been separately reported in recent occupational studies of general cancer incidence and mortality, however, some rather consistent patterns seem to be emerging. In particular, occupational cohorts engaged in a variety of technologically advanced industries are evidencing excesses of MM morbidity and mortality. This is particularly true in cohorts which may be exposed to unusual chemicals or unusual sources of radiation. Interestingly, these excesses are temporally concordant with dramatic increases in MM incidence rates among employment-aged (ages 20-64) men over the last few decades. In the San Francisco Bay area, MM rates for men in these age groups doubled in the decade from 1960 to 1970, doubled again between 1970 and 1980, and are still increasing rapidly (Resource for Cancer Epidemiology, California Dept. of Health Services, unpublished data).

The evidence from the wide gamut of study designs considered here argues strongly for occupational risk factors for MM. There is no one definitive study; the evidence is scattered and plagued by the problem of small numbers. Nonetheless, despite these limitations, the consistencies in these studies allow the formulation of enough hypotheses for us to begin to direct our energies at trying to elucidate these possible risks.

References

Adelstein AM (1972) Occupational mortality: cancer. Ann Occup Hyg 15: 53-57

Armstrong BK, McNulty JC, Levitt LJ, Williams KA, Hobbs MST (1979) Mortality in gold and coal miners in Western Australia with special reference to lung cancer. Br J Ind Med 36: 199-205

Austin DF (1982) Evaluation of the occurrence of malignant melanoma in the Caltrans headquarters building: a report to the department of transportation. Resource for Cancer Epidemiology Emeryville

Austin DF, Reynolds P (1984) A case-control study of malignant melanoma among Lawrence Livermore National Laboratory employees: final report submitted to the LLNL, July 3, 1984. Resource for Cancer Epidemiology, Emeryville

Austin DF, Reynolds PJ (Manscript in preparation) Occupations at increased risk for malignant melanoma of the skin: A proportional incidence analysis.

Austin DF, Reynolds PJ, Synder M, Biggs MW, Stubbs HA (1981) Malignant melanoma among employees of Lawrence Livermore National Laboratory. Lancet 2: 712-716

Bahn AK, Rosenwaike I, Herrmann N, Grover P, Stellman J, O'Leary K (1976) Melanoma after exposure to PCB's. N Engl J Med 295: 450

Beral V, Robinson N (1981) The relationship of malignant melanoma, basal and squamous skin cancers to indoor and outdoor work. Br J Cancer 44: 886-891

Blot WJ, Brinton LA, Fraumeni JF, Stone BS (1977) Cancer mortality in U.S. counties with petroleum industries. Science 198: 51-53

Caldwell GG, Kelley D, Zack M, Falk H, Heath CW (1983) Mortality and cancer frequency among military nuclear test (Smoky) participants, 1957 through 1979. JAMA 250(5): 620-624

Committee for the Cancer-Environment Registry (1980) The Swedish Cancer Environment Registry 1961-1973. National Board of Health and Welfare, Stockholm

Decoufle P, Stanislawczyk K (1977) A retrospective survey of cancer in relation to occupation. DHEW (NIOSH), Cincinnati (Publication no. 77-178)

Dubrow R, Wegman DH (1984) Cancer and occupation in Massachusetts: a death certificate study. Am I Ind Med 6: 207-230

Elashoff R, Hunter TD, Mohilef E (1982) Final report on epidemiology of melanoma, NICHD Contract HD-8-2803. University of California at Los Angeles, Los Angeles

Greene MH, Hoover RH, Eck RL, Fraumeni JF (1979) Cancer mortality among printing plant workers. Environ Res 20: 66-73

Hadjimichael OC, Ostfeld AM, D'Atri DA, Brubaker RE (1983) Mortality and cancer incidence experience of employees in a nuclear fuels fabrication plant. J Occup Med 25 (1): 48-61

Heldaas SS, Langard SL, Andersen A (1984) Incidence of cancer among vinyl chloride and polyvinyl chloride workers. Br J Ind Med 41: 25-30

Hilt B, Langard S, Andersen A, Rosenberg J (to be published). Asbestos exposure, smoking habits and cancer incidence among production and maintenance workers in an electrochemical plant.

Hoar SK, Pell S (1981) A retrospective cohort study of mortality and cancer incidence among chemists. J Occup Med 23 (7): 485-494

Holman CDJ (1982) Risk factors in the causation of human malignant melanoma of the skin. Ph. D. Dissertation, University of Western Australia.

Holmberg B, Westerholm P, Maasing R, Kestrup L, Gumaelius K, Holmlund L, Englund A (1983) Retrospective cohort study of two plants in the Swedish rubber industry. Scand J Work Environ Health 9 [Suppl 2]: 59-68

Hoover R, Fraumeni JF (1975) Cancer mortality in U.S. counties with chemical industries. Environ Res 9: 197-207

Lee JAH, Strickland D (1980) Malignant melanoma: social status and outdoor work. Br J Cancer 41: 757-763

Logan WPD (1982) Cancer mortality by occupation and social class: 1851-1971. IARC Sci Publ 36

Matanoski GM, Seltser R, Sartwell PE, Diamond EL, Elliott EA (1975) The current mortality rates of radiologists and other physician specialists: specific causes of death. Am J Epidemiol 101 (3): 199-210

Milham S (1976) Occupational mortality in Washington State, 1950-1971. DHEW, Cincinnati

Olin R, Vagero D, Ahlbom A (1985) Mortality experience of electrical engineers. Br J Ind Med 42: 211-212

Pell S, O'Berg MT, Karrh BW (1978) Cancer epidemiologic surveillance in the DuPont Company. J Occup Med 20 (11): 725-740

Petersen GR, Milham S (1980) NIOSH research report: occupational mortality in the State of California 1959-1961. National Institute for Occupational Safety and Health, Cincinnati. [DHEW publication no. (NIOSH)80-104]

Rushton L, Alderson MR (1981) An epidemiological survey of eight oil refineries in Britain. Br J Ind Med 38: 225-234

Stellman SD, Garfinkel L (1984) Cancer mortality among woodworkers. Am J Ind Med 5: 343-357

Teppo L, Pukkala E, Hakama M, Hakulinen T, Herva A, Saxen E (1980) Way of life and cancer incidence in Finland. Scand J Soc Med [Suppl 19]

Thomas TL, Decoufle P (1979) Mortality among workers employed in the pharmaceutical industry: a preliminary investigation. J Occup Med 21 (9): 619-623

Thomas TL, Decoufle P, Moure-Eraso R (1980) Mortality among workers employed in petroleum refining and petrochemical plants. J Occup Med 22 (2): 97-103

Vagero D, Olin R (1983) Incidence of cancer in the electronics industry: using the new Swedish Cancer Environment Registry as a screening instrument. Br J Ind Med 40: 188-192

Vagero D, Persson G (1984) Risk, survival and trends of malignant melanoma among white and blue-collar workers in Sweden. Soc Sci Med 19: 475-478

Vagero D, Ahlbom A, Olin R, Sahlsten S (1985) Cancer morbidity among workers in the telecommunications industry. Br J Ind Med 42: 191-195

Waxweiler RJ, Alexander V, Leffingwell SS, Haring ML, Lloyd JW (1983) Mortality from brain tumor and other causes in a cohort of petrochemical workers. INCI 70: 75-81

Williams RR, Stegens HL, Goldsmith JR (1977) Associations of cancer site and type with occupations and industry from the Third National Cancer Survey interview. JNCI 59 (4): 1147-1185

Wright WE, Peters JM, Mack TM (1983) Organic chemicals and malignant melanoma. Am J Ind Med 4 (4): 577-581

Current Issues in Melanoma Research: Exogenous Hormones, Pregnancy

*Cutaneous Melanoma and Oral Contraceptives: A Review of Case-Control and Cohort Studies**, **

E. A. Holly

Northern California Cancer Program, P. O. Box 101 44, Palo Alto, CA 94303, USA

Introduction

There is biological evidence for the hypothesis that the frequency of malignant melanoma is influenced by hormonal or reproductive factors. Estrogen receptors have been found in human malignant melanoma cells, though the percent age that are estrogen positive varies considerably by study (Creagan et al. 1980; Fisher et al. 1976). Estrogens and progesterone together or estrogen alone increase the number of melanocytes and the intracellular and extracellular melanin content in guinea pigs (Snell and Bischitz 1960). Ultraviolet light exposure causes darkening of the skin pigment and is believed to play a role in the etiology of melanoma (Holman and Armstrong 1984). Estrogens, whether administered topically (Jadassohn 1958), used to relieve menopausal symptoms (Hamilton 1939), or taken for contraception, can also produce hyperpigmentation, the degree of darkening increasing with duration of use (Carruthers 1966).

Several studies over the past decade examined the relationship between oral contraceptives (OCs) and melanoma, with various outcomes (Adam et al. 1981; Bain et al. 1982; Beral et al. 1984, 1977; Gallagher et al. 1985; Helmrich et al. 1984; Holly et al. 1983; Holman et al. 1984; Kay 1981; Ramcharan et al. 1981). This paper reviews and compares the results of these studies and mentions other reproductive factors that should be considered in future research.

Review

Table 1 summarizes the studies presented with a distinction made between risk estimates for ever use vs never use of OCs, and long-term use vs short-term or no use. Case-control and cohort studies are presented, each with the publication date. The study population is noted, as is the city or region where the study was conducted. The numbers of cases and controls or the number of women in the cohort or of woman-years are given for each study. When there were other hormone-related factors of interest they also are mentioned.

* The work reported in this paper was supported in part by NCI grants CA 34382 and CA 19408

** *Abbreviations: MM,* malignant melanoma; *SSM,* superficial spreading melanoma; *NM,* nodular melanoma; *OC,* oral contraceptives

Recent Results in Cancer Research. Vol 102

The studies are reviewed in the text in the order published and are separated in the table by study type (case-control or cohort).

Beral and her colleagues reported the results of two small studies of melanoma using data from the Kaiser-Permanente Health Plan in Walnut Creek, California (Beral et al. 1977). The first, a follow-up study of 17,942 women aged 17-59, reported relative risks of 1.4 and 1.7 for melanoma among users of OC for fewer than 4 years and for 4 years or more, respectively, when compared with women who had never used these agents. Twenty-two women were diagnosed as having melanoma during the study period among the 18000 women who entered the study. The authors also reported increased risk associated with ever use of noncontraceptive estrogens, with a relative risk of 1.8. The second study used a case-control design with 37 cases and 74 age-matched controls in women aged 20-59, and estimated the odds ratio of melanoma among ever users of OCs to be 1.8 times that of women who had never used them. The number of cases in each study was small, however, and the associations were not statistically significant.

Ramcharan et al. reported results from a follow-up study conducted in a large California-based health plan (Ramcharan et al. 1981). The relative risk for melanoma for ever use of OCs was 3.5 over all age groups combined (confidence limits (CL) = 1.4-9.0). The study population for this analysis included 16 melanoma cases in a population of 14,104 women aged 18-64 who responded to the 1977 interim questionnaire. Several potentially confounding variables were considered in analysis. The percentage distribution of hours of exposure to sunlight by current, past, or never use of OCs was nearly identical. The number of cases was small and histological type was not considered in the analysis.

Kay reported 40 cases of melanoma through 1979 in the English Royal College of General Practitioners follow-up study of OC use and health (Kay 1981). The relative risk, based on a total of 306,286 woman-years of observation, was 1.5 (CL=0.73-2.9). Kay's brief letter to the editor presented no data on subjects' age, histological diagnosis, or risk by time interval.

Adam et al. (1981) reported an odds ratio of 1.6 for melanoma among women aged 15-49 who had used OCs for 5 years or more compared with the risk among women who had never used these agents (CL=0.83-3.0). The odds ratio for ever use vs never use on their record review study of 158 cases and 503 controls was 1.3 (CL=0.92-1.96). A postal survey of a subset of these women noted an odds ratio of 1.1 (CL=0.73-1.8). No potentially confounding variables were noted in this study of English women. No analyses by histological subcategories of melanoma were included.

In a postal survey of registered nurses in 11 states in the United States of America, no overall relationship between melanoma and OC use was observed in 141 women with melanoma and 2,820 age-matched nurses without this disease (Bain et al. 1982). Elevated odds ratios for use of these agents were noted for women who were less than age 40 at diagnosis in this population of women ages 30-55 years. The risk estimate for these women was 1.4 (CL=0.83-2.46) when adjusted for geography, parity, age at first pregnancy, height and prior hair dye use. Univariate odds ratios were 1.4 for women who had used OCs for 1-24 months (CL=0.71-2.6) and 2.3 (CL=1.3-4.0) for those who had used them for 25 months or more. However, adjustment for the above-mentioned variables diminished the magnitude of these associations to 1.2 and 1.7, and the risk estimate for longer use was no longer statistically significant. Women less than age 40 who used OCs for at least 2 years beginning 10 or more years before diagnosis had a crude odds ratio of 3.0 (CL=1.16-7.49). Multivariate analysis reduced this estimate to 2.3 (CL=0.77-6.94). In the much smaller group of women over age 40 no association with use of OCs was noted. The information available was inadequate for analysis by histological type.

Table 1. Summary of results of studies of melanoma and oral contraceptive use

Literature reference study population, location	No. of cases, no. of controls, or no. in cohort	Relative risk estimates for oral contraceptive use		Other hormone-related factors of interest	Comments
		Ever use vs never use	Long-term use[c] vs short-term use or no use		
Case-control					
Beral et al. 1977 Kaiser Health Plan Controls randomly chosen by age from same plan, California	37 74	1.8	No data	-	Information on sunlight exposure, complexion, etc. not available. Small numbers prevented subgroup analysis
Adam et al. 1981 Population-based record review, postal survey, Oxford[a]	158 503	1.1 1.3	1.6	-	OC was not related to any risk factors for melanoma, personal characteristics were considered
Bain et al. 1982 Postal survey of registered nurses in 11 states in U.S.	141 2,820	0.9	2.3 3.0*	-	Adjustment made for geographic area. Direct control for exposure to sunlight, skin color and histological type not possible
Holly et al. 1983 Population-based cases and controls, Seattle	87 863	1.2	2.4* 3.6* 4.4* 5.1*	Association between melanoma and age at birth of first child at 31+ years*	Information on sunlight exposure, complexion, etc. not available. Risk by time interval was assessed
Helmrich et al. 1984 Hospital based, Boston	160 640	0.9	1.0 1.2 1.1 0.7		Hospitalized cases may have been a select group; hospitalized controls may have used OCs at higher rate than general population. Information on sunlight exposure, complexion, histology, etc., not available
Beral et al. 1984 Melanoma clinic population controls 74%, hospital controls 26%, Sydney, Australia	287 574	1.0	1.5*	Association between melanoma and use of hormones to regulate periods; for menopausal use; and	Controlled for exposure to sunlight, complexion, and other variables. Risk by time interval was assessed

Holman et al. 1984 Population-based cases Controls from registered voters and public school, Western Australia	276 276	1.0	1.1 1.6 4.7	Borderline association between melanoma and use of menopausal estrogens	Controlled for exposure to sunlight, complexion and other variables. Risk by time interval was assessed
Gallagher et al. 1985 Population-based cases and controls, W. Canada	361 361	1.0	0.9	Association between lowered incidence of melanoma and higher no. of live births* and between lowered incidence of melanoma and bilateral oophorectomy*	controlled for exposure to sunlight, complexion and other variables. Risk by time interval was assessed
Cohort					
Beral et al. 1977 Kaiser Health Plan, Calif.	22 17,942	1.4	1.7	Association between melanoma and ever use of estrogens other than OC use	Information on sunlight exposure, complexion, etc. not available. Small numbers prevented subgroup analysis
Ramcharan et al. 1981 Kaiser Health Plan, Calif.	16 14,104	3.5*	No data	–	Melanoma-OC use association persisted after consideration of other factors. OC use not associated with exposure to sunlight
Kay 1981 Royal College of General Practitioners, UK	40 306,286[b]	1.5	No data	–	Brief letter to the editor, no mention of exposure to sunlight, complexion, or risk by time interval

[a] 1.1 from postal survey, 1.3 from medical record review

[b] Woman-years of observation

[c] Long-term use definitions: Beral et al. (1977), 4+ years; Adam et al. (1981), 5+ years; Bain et al. (1982), 2+ years beginning 10+ years before diagnosis, women age 40, multivariate analysis, univariate; Holly et al. (1983), 5–9 years; 10+ years; 5+ years use first beginning 12+ years before diagnosis; 5+ years use with at least 5 years since last use for SSM only; Helmrich et al. (1984), 5+ years beginning 10+ years before diagnosis, all cases; 5+ years Clark levels I and II; III; and IV and V, respectively; Beral et al. (1984), 5+ years beginning 10+ years before diagnosis; Holman et al. (1984), all melanomas 5+ years use; SSM 5+ years use; Hutchinson melanotic freckle 2+ years, respectively; Gallagher et al. (1985), 5+ years

* Significantly different from 1 ($P<0.05$)

A population-based study of 87 women with melanoma and 863 randomly chosen controls in women aged 37-74 conducted in Seattle and the surrounding county in Washington State noted no overall association between all histological types of melanoma and OC use (Holly et al. 1983). However, for superficial spreading melanoma (SSM) odds ratios for users of OCs for 5-9 and 10 years or more were 2.4 and 3.6, respectively (P value for trend = 0.004). No differences between cases and controls were noted for OC use of 4 years or less. The women at greatest risk of being diagnosed as having SSM were those who took OCs for at least 5 years starting 12 or more years before diagnosis, for whom the odds ratio was 4.4 (CL = 2.0-9.7), and those who took them for at least 5 years ending 5 or more years before diagnosis, for whom the odds ratio was 5.1 (CL = 2.0-12.8). These elevated odds ratios may indicate the effects of a longer latent period or the stronger dose pill used in the 1960s. Only women who were in an age group that could have used OCs (37-59 years) were considered for these analyses. Giving birth to a first child after age 30 was also associated with an elevated risk of SSM. No other reproductive factors of the several considered, including menopausal estrogen use, were found to be a risk factor for any form of melanoma. The findings of the Seattle study make clear the need for subgroup analysis by histological type.

No statistically significant association between OC use and melanoma was found in a Boston University study of 160 hospitalized melanoma patients and 640 hospitalized controls aged 20-59 (Helmrich et al. 1984). No association was noted between melanoma and OCs by duration of use or by years since first and last use. Pathology reports available for some cases were categorized for Clark level of tumor thickness. Clark levels I and II are more likely to include a greater proportion of SSM than Clark levels IV and V, though other histological tumor types are likely to be included in all Clark level groups. Relative risk estimates were 1.2 for levels I and II, 1.1 for level III, and 0.7 for levels IV and V for OC use of 5 or more years' duration. Adequate information was not available for analysis by histological subtype.

Beral et al. (1984), in a study conducted in Sydney, Australia among women ages 18-54, noted no increased risk for melanoma among OC users when all use groups were considered together. In their study of 287 women with melanoma and 574 mostly population-based controls (about 25% hospital-based controls were included in this group), they observed an elevated risk of MM of 1.5 (CL = 1.03-2.14) among women who had taken OCs for at least 5 years starting 10 or more years prior to diagnosis. After adjusting for numerous potentially confounding factors, odds ratios for women who had taken OCs remained essentially the same and the results were statistically significant. Elevated odds ratios also were noted for other forms of female sex hormones - use of hormones to regulate periods (odds ratio = 1.9); hormone replacement therapy (1.4); and use of hormonal injections to suppress lactation (1.4). Numbers were small in each of these groups and the elevated estimates did not differ statistically from one. No statistically significant differences were noted by histological subtype for OC use.

A study recently completed by Holman et al. (1984) in Western Australia among females aged 10-79 years showed no statistically significant relationship between any histological subtype of melanoma and OC use among 276 cases and 276 controls. The odds ratios for SSM, with numerous potential confounding factors considered in analysis, were 0.78 (CL = 0.32-1.9) for women using OCs for less than 2 years, 2.2 (CL = 0.73-6.8) for 2-4 years of use, and 1.6 (CL = 0.53-4.9) for a history of 5 or more years of use. The relationship between OCs and specific subtypes of melanoma was also considered by time period in an attempt to assess latency. Numbers in these subgroups were necessarily small and there were no statistically significant findings.

Odds ratios were 1.3 for SSM and 2.5 for Hutchinson's melanotic freckle for ever use of OC 10 or more years before diagnosis. Borderline evidence of an association between SSM and duration of use of unopposed estrogens was noted in this study: odds ratios for 1–12 months of use and 13+ months were 1.7 and 2.3, respectively (P value for trend = 0.08).

A recent study by Gallagher et al. revealed no increased risk for ever use of OC and no increased risk by histological subtype. When age groups 20–39 and 40–69 were analyzed separately no increased risk for use of OC was noted in either group. Women who had five or more children were at a decreased risk of melanoma (odds ratio = 0.4, $P = 0.02$), as were women who had had a bilateral oophorectomy (odds ratio = 0.5, $P = 0.02$). Sunlight exposure was considered in this study and no relationship was noted with OC use.

Discussion

Overall, when all age, histological types, and OC use groups are considered together, there appears to be at best a modest effect of OC on melanoma. Only the follow-up study by Ramcharan et al. showed strong evidence of an association between ever use of OCs and risk for all histological types of melanoma. Holman et al. (1984), after calculating a weighted average of estimates of risk from seven studies, suggested that if *ever use* of OCs is a risk factor for melanoma, the overall increased risk due to these substances is no more than one-third above that of women who have never used OC. To test the hypothesis that there is no association between ever use of OC and melanoma, we used the sign test (Siegel 1956). Studies that had odds ratios or relative risks < 1.0 for melanoma–OC associations that were counted as negative and those with values > 1.0, as positive, with 1.0 values dropped from consideration. There were six studies with positive relative risks or odds ratios and two negative odds ratios ($P = 0.15$). The sign test indicates that there is probably little effect, if any, for ever use of OCs.

The concern about an effect of OCs becomes more troublesome when subgroup analyses are considered. The long-term use definitions are all different for the studies reviewed here, making it difficult to compare results directly. Small samples in the subgroups have not generated statistically significant elevated odds ratios for many studies for long-term OC users. For this reason the sign test was used again. For long-term use vs no use or short-term use, there were one negative and seven positive odds ratios or relative risk estimates with a P value of 0.04. The sign test indicates that we may not be able to dismiss a possible association between melanoma and long-term OC use too casually.

To sort out complex relationships among variables, future research conducted on the effects of endogenous and exogenous estrogens on melanoma must consider:

- Case and control group selection
- The possible different effects OCs may have on histological types of melanoma
- Age, stronger dose pill used in the 1960s, latency and duration of use by time period
- Other potential confounders, such as sunlight
- Other reproductive factors

Large samples are necessary, and subgroup analyses have to be carefully planned to minimize problems with multiple comparisons. These factors and others are briefly discussed below.

Case and Control Group Selection

A population-based study best avoids selective case ascertainment in the study of melanoma and the problems inherent in studies using hospital or neighborhood controls. For the study of most cancers, hospitalized cases do not necessarily present a problem. However, the vast majority of melanoma patients, particularly those with SSM, are diagnosed and managed as outpatients for their primary tumor. Thus, a study using only hospitalized patients could have a highly select case population and perhaps a larger proportion of patients with nodular melanoma (NM) than would be found in a population-based study. To date, there have been no elevated odds ratios associated with long-term OC use and NM in any of the studies that have considered histologic type.

Control group selection may be an important factor in the study of melanoma and OC use. Use of a hospitalized control group could underestimate the strength of any association between OC use and melanoma. In support of this concern, a study of 66,000 women conducted by a group from the Department of Epidemiology at Harvard University reported that women who took OCs in the Boston area had a 20% or greater increase in hospitalization rates than nonusers (Hoover et al. 1978). This increase occurred even for conditions *unlikely* to be related biologically to OC use. They gave specific examples of trauma and appendectomy. These two groups made up nearly 50% of the Boston University (Helmrich et al. 1984) control group population.

Neighborhood controls may present another problem, in that persons of like socioeconomic status tend to have similar health habits and live in similar neighborhoods. Since the use of OCs varies with social and reproductive factors (Hoover et al. 1978), use of neighborhood controls may overmatch on OC use and other variables of interest.

Histological Type

The studies reviewed here and other evidence (Holman and Armstrong 1984) indicate the importance of conducting analyses by histological type. When all age groups, histological types, and OC use groups were considered together, few etiologic clues were noted and the overall risk of melanoma from OC use, if it exists, was minimal. While random fluctuation is likely to be partially responsible, SSM and NM appeared to present enough of a different picture to warrant separate analysis. Because the patients with NM were so few in the studies reviewed here no data have been presented on this subtype. Though the numbers were quite small in the four studies that considered NM, this tumor type often had odds ratios in the opposite direction to those for SSM, particularly when long-term OC use was considered [Gallagher et al. 1985; Helmrich et al. 1984 (if Clark levels IV and V are used as rough indicators for NM); Holly et al. 1983 (unpublished data); Holman et al. 1984].

While there was no hint of statistical significance in the studies just mentioned, some effort should be made to look for etiologic clues in a large series of patients who have been diagnosed as having NM. If a statistically significant opposite effect for NM and OC use occurs in larger series of this tumor type, some thought must be given to personal or sociologic characteristics that might explain why women who are diagnosed as having NM have not taken OCs in the same proportion as have controls.

Age, OC Dose, Latency, Duration of Use by Time Period

Young women today have not had the opportunity to use OCs over a long time period, nor have they been exposed to the stronger dose pill available in the 1960s. Thus, they first should be considered separately from women aged 35–55, who may have taken OCs in the stronger doses in the 1960s and have perhaps taken OCs for a longer time period. In contrast, women aged 60–79 at diagnosis would have been either postmenopausal in the 1960s or in an age group that would not have commonly used OCs and so should not be included in the OC analyses. The same policy should apply for menopausal estrogens. That is, only women who were in an age group eligible to use menopausal estrogens should be included in the analysis of an association between melanoma and use of these preparations. Age groups in each of the studies reviewed were analyzed differently. Some studies considered all age groups together, while others either age-adjusted their results or did age-specific subgroup analyses.

Within the appropriate age groups, careful attention should be paid to whether women used the stronger dose pill. Actual dosage is often difficult to determine. While women could remember the number of years they took OCs, they were less likely to remember *when* they took a particular brand, especially if they took them years ago and used several brands. Thus, it is nearly impossible to assess dosage accurately. An estimate of the dosage effect can be achieved by considering the time period when the women used OC, since the preparations available in 1962 were, in general, much stronger than those commonly used in 1982. Dose, duration of use by time period, and latency can be estimated together by considering, for example, only women who had taken OCs for at least 5 years and who began to take them at least 10 or 15 years ago.

Other combinations that take into account age, dose, duration by time period, and latency can be considered, depending upon the number of women under study who have been diagnosed as having melanoma. Detailed subgroup analyses require sample sizes found only in the largest of studies. This is one of the more difficult problems inherent in the study of melanoma and use of OCs. Future studies should be large enough to permit adequate subgroup analyses.

Sunlight and Other Potential Confounders

Effects of OC and other reproductive factors may be modified in geographic areas with very intense sunlight and high incidence rates of melanoma. Variation in exposure to sunlight may partially explain differences between results in studies from areas of low and high exposure such as Seattle, Vancouver, and Australia. Exposure to sunlight was not measured in several studies reviewed here and may have been a confounding factor, though it was unrelated to OC use in the melanoma studies conducted in California (Ramcharan et al. 1981), Oxford, England (Adam et al. 1981), and Western Canada (Gallagher et al. 1985).

Other Reproductive Factors

Three studies noted elevated risks for use of replacement estrogens though no statistically significant associations were found (Beral et al. 1977, 1984; Holman et al. 1984). Individual studies reported statistically significant associations between melanoma and assorted reproductive factors - age at birth of first child at 31 years or older was noted as a risk factor in one study (Holly et al. 1983); a decrease in melanoma risk was noted for women with greater numbers of live births; and a decrease in risk was noted for women who had had bilateral oophorectomies (Gallagher et al. 1985). Two other studies also reported decreased risks with five or more children, though they were not statistically significant (Holly et al. 1983; Holman et al. 1984). An increase in melanoma risk for women who used hormones to regulate their periods or to stop lactation, though not statistically significant, was noted in another study (Beral et al. 1984). Most of the variables just mentioned have been considered in only two, or at the most three, separate studies. Each of these factors should be considered in any future research on melanoma and reproductive factors.

Future Directions

A simple picture cannot be drawn for melanoma and a possible association between either exogenous or endogenous estrogens. It is somewhat reassuring to know that there does not appear to be an increased risk of melanoma for the vast majority of women who have ever used OCs. However, the results are more disturbing when long-term use of OCs, duration and time of use, and histology are considered. Many variables discussed in this presentation were not statistically significant and therefore were not *technically* related to melanoma. They are presented here as clues to the primary areas that should be considered in future studies of melanoma and endogenous and exogenous hormones. Other variables thought to be related to hormone-dependent cancers (e.g., breast and ovary) should also be considered.

There is a need for more large, carefully designed and carefully analyzed population-based studies to address the unresolved issues outlined above. Currently, two large studies are under way in California to consider the effects of endogenous and exogenous estrogens on melanoma; both use population-based cases, one with neighborhood controls and the other with population-based controls.

References

Adam SA, Sheaves JK, Wright NH, Mosser RW, Vessey MP (1981) A case-control study of the possible association between oral contraceptives and malignant melanoma. Br J Cancer 44: 45-50

Bain C, Hennekens CH, Speizer FE, Rosner B, Willett W, Belanger C (1982) Oral contraceptive use and malignant melanoma. JNC I 68: 537-539

Beral V, Ramcharan S, Faris R (1977) Malignant melanoma and oral contraceptive use among women in California. Br J Cancer 36: 804-809

Beral V, Evans S, Shaw H, Milton G (1984) Oral contraceptive use and malignant melanoma in Australia. Br J Cancer 50: 681-685

Carruthers R (1966) Chloasma and oral contraceptives. Med J Aust 2: 17-20

Creagan ET, Ingle JN, Woods JE, Pritchard DJ, Jiang NS (1980) Estrogen receptors in patients with malignant melanoma. Cancer 46: 1785-1786

Fisher RI, Neifeld JP, Lippman ME (1976) Oestrogen receptors in human malignant melanoma. Lancet 2: 337-338

Gallagher RP, Elwood JM, Hill GB, Coldman AJ, Threlfall WJ, Spinelli JJ (1985) Reproductive factors, oral contraceptives and risk of malignant melanoma: Western Canada melanoma study. Br J Cancer 52: 901-907

Hamilton JB (1939) Significance of sex hormones in tanning of the skin of women. Proc Soc Exp Biol Med 40: 402-503

Helmrich SP, Rosenberg L, Kaufman DW, Miller DR, Schottenfeld D, Stolley PD, Shapiro S (1984) Lack of an elevated risk of malignant melanoma in relation to oral contraceptive use. JNCI 72: 617-620

Holly EA, Weiss NS, Liff JM (1983) Cutaneous melanoma in relation to exogenous hormones and reproductive factors. JNCI 70: 827-831

Holman CDJ, Armstrong BK (1984) Cutaneous malignant melanoma and indicators of total accumulated exposure to the sun: an analysis separating histogenetic types. JNCI 73: 75-82

Holman CDJ, Armstrong BK, Heenan PJ (1984) Cutaneous malignant melanoma in women: exogenous sex hormones and reproductive factors. Br J Cancer 50: 673-680

Hoover R, Bain C, Cole P, MacMahon B (1978) Oral contraceptive use: association with frequency of hospitalization and chronic disease risk indicators. Am J Public Health 68: 335-341

Jadassohn W (1958) Art for art's sake in medicine. Arch Dermatol 78: 427-437

Kay CR (1981) (letter) Malignant melanoma and oral contraceptives. Br J Cancer 44: 479

Ramcharan S, Pellegrin FA, Ray R, Hsu JP (1981) The Walnut Creek contraceptive drug study. A prospective study of the side effects of oral contraceptives, vol III. US Government Printing Office, Washington D.C.

Siegel S (1956) Nonparametric statistics. McGraw-Hill, New York, pp 68-75

Snell RS, Bischitz PG (1960) The effect of large doses of estrogen and estrogen and progesterone on melanin pigmentation. J Invest Dermatol 35: 73-82

Melanoma and Pregnancy[*], [**]

E. A. Holly

Northern California Cancer Program, P. O. Box 10144, Palo Alto, CA 94303, USA

Introduction

Pregnancy and its dramatic increase in endogenous hormones may affect malignant melanoma (MM), either through initiation or promotion of a lesion or by affecting prognosis. There is physiological evidence that endogenous and exogenous hormones can affect pigmentation, and animal experiments have shown estrogens to promote tumor growth. This evidence originates from several areas:

- Pregnancy is normally associated with pigment deposition in areas already pigmented and occasionally results in hyperpigmentation of the face.
- Melanocyte-stimulating hormone rises progessively throughout pregnancy with its highest concentration at term (Ances and Pomerantz 1974).
- Steroid hormone receptors have been found in human melanomas (Neifeld and Lippman 1980; Grill et al. 1982).
- Exogenous hormones, primarily oral contraceptives, have been shown to be associated with melasma and the magnitude of this effect increases with duration of use of these agents (Carruthers 1966).
- Experiments with mice have shown an increase in melanoma tumor size upon administration of estrogens in both male and female animals (Lopez et al. 1978).
- Some studies have reported an association between the long-term use of oral contraceptives prior to being diagnosed as having MM (Bain et al. 1982; Holly et al. 1983; Beral et al. 1984), indicating that exogenous hormones may play a role.

Because of this diverse evidence linking hormones and pigmentation, and estrogens and tumor growth, questions arise as to whether pregnancy with its increase in hormones and pigment changes may initiate growth of a melanoma, or whether a pregnancy coincident with MM may affect survival. The negative effects of pregnancy on MM have been the subject of many reports. Case reports and patient series brought attention to the rapidly fatal outcome sometimes observed in pregnant women with melanoma (Lerner et al. 1979; Pack and Scharnagel 1951; Sutherland et al. 1983). There have also been reports of

* The work reported in this paper was supported in part by NCI grants CA 34382 and CA 19408 to the Northern California Cancer Program

** *Abbreviation: MM,* malignant melanoma

Recent Results in Cancer Research. Vol 102

regression of the disease at delivery (Allen 1955; Pennington 1983). Several studies followed early case reports in an attempt at improving understanding of the relationship between pregnancy and melanoma prognosis.

Studies to Date

The published studies that have generally quantified an association between pregnancy and melanoma are summarized in Table 1, which gives a literature reference for each study and its outcome, the number of subjects in each comparison group, and the geographic areas where the studies were conducted. A separate column in the table clarifies the definitions of pregnancy-associated MM if necessary. Finally, results and comments are briefly presented.

The 11 studies included in Table 1 showed essentially no survival difference between the women with MM that was somehow associated with pregnancy and those with MM with no pregnancy association, despite the diverse ways of defining the groups of pregnant women.

Definition of Pregnancy Groups

One of the primary problems with several of the studies reviewed here is the mixing of events that may or may not be related to the prognosis of women with MM. This problem was manifested in some studies by combining women who had been pregnant years before their diagnosis of MM with those pregnant at time of diagnosis, or after diagnosis of MM. Could a pregnancy that occurred 20 years before the diagnosis of a melanoma have any effect on the prognosis of that disease? Perhaps, if sensitization to fetal antigens (Hersey et al. 1977), as discussed below, does occur. It would be difficult to detect an adverse effect of concurrent pregnancy and MM if only a small subset of women with MM were affected. This would be true particularly if these women were combined with those who had been pregnant up to 20 and 30 years before. Thus some of the studies may not have been able to detect any existing association.

In the studies reviewed here, some workers used population-based incidence or mortality data and considered marital status as an indirect indicator of parity (Lee and Hill 1970; Weiss and Flannery 1978). The others were based on chart reviews with considerable variation in pregnancy group definitions.

Primary Question Considered in the 11 Reports

The question considered most often was:
Is survival adversely affected if MM is somehow related to pregnancy?

Of the 11 studies reviewed, 10 showed no survival difference between women whose melanoma was in some way related to a pregnancy and those for whom there was no pregnancy association (see Table 1).

One of the 11 studies noted that pregnant women in one of their subgroups, those with stage II disease, had a poorer survival than the control group (Shiu et al. 1976).

Another group reported better survival for women who had previously been pregnant (Hersey et al. 1977). The authors hypothesized that the apparent protective effect of preg-

Table 1. Malignant melanoma (MM) and pregnancy

Reference MM-Pregnancy Association[a]	Patient population, study type, location	MM–Pregnancy classification	Results	Comments
George et al. (1960) [a]	A. 115 women with MM, pregnancy associated with disease B. 330 women with MM, pregnancy not associated (Chart review in NYC, 1917–1957)	A. 77 women were pregnant when they were diagnosed as having MM. 38 women became pregnant after the definitive treatment of their MM. No time was given as to how long between diagnosis of MM and the subsequent pregnancy B. 330 women not pregnant during the clinical course of the MM. 144 of these women were the same age as group A (16–43 years)	Women who had melanoma associated with pregnancy presented at a later stage[b] 5- and 10-year survival approximately the same in both groups	Stage of disease and age were considered
White et al. (1961) [a]	A. 30 women pregnant within 6 years of their diagnosis of MM B. 31 not pregnant near the diagnosis of MM C. 10 pregnancy undetermined, from a chart review CA tumor registry & Stanford	A. 30 women who were pregnant 1 year before, during or within 5 years after, their diagnosis with MM Number in each of the three subgroups was not given B. 31 women who were not pregnant in this 6-year period C. 10 women for whom no record of pregnancy could be found	Pregnant patients presented at an earlier stage 5-year survival the same No difference in survival time whether MM diagnosis was made before, during or after pregnancy Same proportion of women in each group had rapid spread and early death	Pregnant group had better survival until stage of disease and age were controlled Pregnant women may have had earlier diagnosis of MM as a result of MD visits The women most ill after diagnosis perhaps did not become pregnant

Lee and Hill (1970) a	A. 1943 married women B. 332 single women (Registry data, England and Wales, 1959–1967)	A. 1943 women who were listed as married when they were diagnosed as having MM B. 332 women who were listed as single when they were diagnosed as having MM. No mention was made of divorced or widowed women	Age-specific death rates for MM did not differ by marital status	Marital status used as indirect measure of parity Birth rates for both single and married women were presented and varied considerably by age
Shiu et al. (1976)	A. 47 nulliparous women B, C, D.204 parous women	A. 47 nulliparous women with MM B. 134 parous women with no activation of MM during previous pregnancy	Stage I, no difference in survival Stage II, groups C and D had worse survival than A and B	Pregnant women more likely to have lesions on the trunk and symptomatic lesions (groups C and D combined)
Shiu et al. (1976) 0 Stage 1 - Stage 2	(Chart review in New York City, 1950–1969)	C. 36 parous women with activation of MM during previous pregnancy D. 34 women admitted and treated for MM during pregnancy	20% of nulliparous and parous groups were stage II Parous women with previous MM activation during pregnancy had worse survival[b]	Symptomatic lesions not related to survival
Hersey et al. (1977) †	A. 330 previously pregnant, MM patients B. 113 not previously pregnant MM patients (Chart review, Sydney, Australia, 1961–1971)	A. 330 previously pregnant women diagnosed as having MM of whom 65% were under 50 years old B. 113 women with no pregnancies, 72% of whom were under 50 years old	Previously pregnant women had better survival Equal percentage with stages I, II, III in both groups Survival better for previously pregnant women over age 50[b]	Authors suggest immune response to tumors important in preventing dissemination, not in prevention of primary MM lesions
Weiss and Flannery (1978) a	A. 1441 ever married MM patients B. 244 never married MM patients Population-based study (CT tumor registry data, 1935–1975)		No difference in survival between groups at 3 or 5 years Incidence rates for both groups were the same Survival for men same as for women by marital status	Marital status used as an indirect measure of parity Consideration of never married women bearing children and the reverse was made with little change in survival

Table 1. *(continued)*

Reference MM-Pregnancy Association[a]	Patient population, study type, location	MM-Pregnancy classification	Results	Comments
Elwood and Coldman (1978) a	254 ever pregnant MM patients 51 never pregnant MM patients (Vancouver, BC, 1960–1976)		No difference in survival between groups	Restriction of series to cutaneous lesions yielded no difference between groups With adjustment for stage there was no difference between groups
Shaw et al. (1978) a	A. 480 women pregnant prior to MM dx B. 303 women not pregnant prior to MM C. 17 pregnant at dx with MM (Chart review, Sydney, Australia, 1950–1976)	A. Time between pregnancy and diagnosis was not stated B. Nulliparous women prior to diagnosis of MM, may have been pregnant after diagnosis C. No statistics were given to compare this group with the other two	No difference in 5-year survival between groups A and B Clinical stage of melanoma and primary lesion sites were similar to those pregnant at diagnosis and those pregnant before diagnosis	No difference in site of lesions by pregnancy status
Rampen and Mulder (1980) a	Study of survival differences by sex in pts with metastatic melanoma and between parous and nulliparous women 146 women with MM (Chart review, Rotterdam, 1956–1978)	146 women with metastatic melanoma were divided into parous and nulliparous for comparison of survival between groups (no numbers given)	"... survivals for nulliparous and parous women were identical" Survival for women better than for men	Data were not presented for parous and nulliparous women Authors state results support theory of MM being an androgen-dependent tumor and may explain rapid tumor progression with pregnancy and regression at delivery
Houghton et al. (1981) a	12 pregnant at diagnosis 24 not pregnant at diagnosis matched for site and stage to 12 above		Pregnant women (using controls not matched for site and stage) had a poorer survival	Trunk lesions more common in pregnant women

	175 not pregnant at diagnosis Population-based study (Chart review, CT tumor registry, 1950–1954, 1960–1964, 1970–1974)		No difference in survival when matched for site and stage. 13.3 pregnancies expected, 12 observed based on CT birth rates	
Sutherland et al. (1983 a)	A. 18 women pregnant on diagnosis or with MM arising during pregnancy B. 12 women pregnant after diagnosis	A. Patients diagnosed as having MM during pregnancy; MM arose during pregnancy, or was clearly documented as stimulated by pregnancy	"... subsequent pregnancy has little, if any, adverse effect upon melanoma as to activation of the disease"	No statistics presented Groups not really comparable, as those pregnant after diagnosis have already survived an interval before becoming pregnant
Sutherland et al. (1983 b) a	(Chart review, New Orleans, 1957–1983)	B. Patients with no initiation, diagnosis, or stimulation of melanoma during pregnancy who became pregnant 2–96 months after a MM was diagnosed		Site of lesions same in both groups

[a] MM-Pregnancy association: indicates outcome of the study, where 0 = no effect of MM on pregnancy; – = pregnant women did worse; + = previously pregnant women did better

[b] $P \leqslant 0.05$

nancy might be due to sensitization to fetal antigens during pregnancy. The sensitization may create antibodies to help inhibit progression of the melanoma and enhance survival. Their theory is based on the presence of fetal antigens on melanoma cells and immunization against these fetal antigens during pregnancy. However, this study was the only one that showed previously pregnant women to have a longer survival.

One study examined survival separately for women who became pregnant *after* being diagnosed as having MM and compared them with women who did not become pregnant after their diagnosis (Sutherland et al. 1983b). They noted no difference in survival between the groups. Five other reports (George et al. 1960; White et al. 1961; Shiu et al. 1976; Hersey et al. 1977; Shaw et al. 1978) included women who became pregnant after they had been diagnosed as having melanoma, as part of their larger group of pregnancy-associated melanomas. There were no differences in survival between the mixed groups in these five reports, though data were not presented to address the specific subgroup examined by Sutherland et al.

Sex Differences in Incidence and Survival

National cancer data sets show incidence rates among women in the reproductive years to be much higher than among men. Men have higher rates than women in the years after menopause (SEER, 1981). Logically, this indicates support for a hormonally induced cancer hypothesis. Though women have a higher incidence of MM than do men during the early part of their lives, most studies show women with MM to survive longer than men with MM (Shaw et al. 1978; Cancer Patient Survival 1976; Blois et al. 1983). Part of this survival difference can be attributed to women generally having thinner lesions at diagnosis even within Clark's tumor level (Blois et al. 1983). Women also are more likely to have prognostically more favorable lesions on their extremities, while men have prognostically less favorable lesions on their trunk and head and neck (Blois et al. 1983; Shaw et al. 1978). However, women have better survival than men even after adjustment for site, level, and thickness (Blois et al. 1983). Both the incidence patterns and survival data support some hormonal effect on MM, though from the evidence to date, it appears unlikely that pregnancy has a role in overall survival.

Site of Lesion

How the incidence and survival data might be related to hormones in pregnancy is unclear. Perhaps hormones play an adverse role in MM in only a subset of women who are particularly sensitive to their effects. While most studies did not mention site, 2 of the 11 noted that pregnant women were more likely to have prognostically less favorable trunk lesions (Shiu et al. 1976; Houghton et al. 1981). One of these reported a poorer survival for pregnant women when site and stage were not matched. However, this difference disappeared with control for these factors (Houghton et al. 1981). In another report, site did not differ between 17 women who were pregnant when they were diagnosed as having MM, and the other women in the study (Shaw et al. 1978). White et al. also noted no difference by site between their groups, though their pregnant group was not limited to women pregnant only at diagnosis. Whether site of the MM is related to difference in hormonal factors between men and women or to other etiologic factors is unknown.

Characteristics of Women Adversely Affected

Few clues as to characteristics of particular women with MM who may be adversely affected by pregnancy have come from the studies completed to date. It is difficult to determine a profile of these women, since melanoma is a relatively rare disease and pregnancy is normally a 9-months event that occurs infrequently over a woman's lifetime. A primary diagnosis of MM and pregnancy seldom coincide. One study noted that more symptomatic lesions were associated with pregnancy, but no correlation with survival was found (Shiu et al. 1976). Other than symptomatic lesions and the conflicting evidence about lesion site, little information is available to characterize women who are diagnosed as having MM while pregnant.

Comparison of the hormone profiles of women who are affected by their pregnancy with those of other women who have had no pregnancy-MM association may help characterize affected women. These hormonal profiles should be carried out both during and after gestation. Profiles of healthy women without MM would serve as a useful control group.

The 11 studies presented here indicate few, if any, deleterious effects of pregnancy on the survival of the majority of women who have been diagnosed as having MM. While case reports do document rapid spread and early death for some pregnant women, 5-year survival rates of the group of patients as a whole minimize these dramatic cases by including them in the overall statistics. Though rapidly fatal, widespread metastases are seen both in women who are not pregnant and in men, the occurrence in pregnant women tends to be publicized more than similar cases among nonpregnant women or men.

References

Allen EP (1955) Malignant melanoma: spontaneous regression after pregnancy. Br Med J 2: 1067

Ances IG, Pomerantz SH (1974) Serum concentrations of β-melanocyte-stimulating hormone in human pregnancy. Am J Obstet Gynecol 119: 1062-1068

Bain C, Hennekins CH, Speizer FE, Rosner B, Willett W, Belanger C (1982) Oral contraceptive use and malignant melanoma. JNCI 68: 537-539

Beral V, Evans S, Shaw H, Milton G (1984) Oral contraceptive use and malignant melanoma in Austrália. Br J Cancer 50: 681-685

Blois MS, Sagebiel RW, Abarbanel RM, Caldwell TM, Tuttle MS (1983) Malignant melanoma of the skin: I. The association of tumor depth and type, and patient sex, age, and site with survival. Cancer 52: 1330-1341

Carruthers R (1966) Chloasma and oral contraceptives. Med J Aust 2: 17-20

Department of Health, Education, and Welfare (1976) Cancer patients survival. DHEW, Washington (Report no. 5; DHEW publication no. (NIH) 77-992

Department of Health, Education, and Welfare (1981) Surveillance, epidemiology and end results: incidence and mortality data. DHEW, Washington, pp 98-100 (NCI monograph no. 57; DHEW publication no. 81-2330)

Elwood JM, Coldman AJ (1978) Previous pregnancy and melanoma prognosis. Lancet 2: 1000-1001

George PA, Fortner JG, Pack GT (1960) Melanoma with pregnancy: A report of 115 cases. Cancer 13: 854-859

Grill H-J, Benes P, Manz B, et al. (1982) Steroid hormone receptor analysis in human melanoma and non-malignant human skin. Br J Dermatol 107 [Suppl 23]: 64-65

Hersey P, Morgan G, Stone DE, McCarthy WH, Milton GW (1977) Previous pregnancy as a protective factor against death from melanoma. Lancet 1: 451-452

Holly EA, Weiss NS, Liff JM (1983) Cutaneous melanoma in relation to exogenous hormones and reproductive factors. JNCI 70: 827-831
Houghton AN, Flannery J, Viola MV (1981) Malignant melanoma of the skin occurring during pregnancy. Cancer 48: 407-410
Lee JAH, Hill GB (1970) Marriage and fatal malignant melanoma in females. Am J Epidemiol 91: 48-51
Lerner AB, Nordlund JJ, Kirkwood JM (1979) Effects of oral contraceptives and pregnancy on melanomas. (Letter) N Engl J Med 301: 47
Lopez RE, Bhakoo H, Paolini NS, Rosen F, Holyoke ED, Godrosen MH (1978) Effect of estrogen on the growth of B-16 melanoma. Surg Forum 29: 153-154
Neifeld JP, Lippman ME (1980) Seroid hormone receptors and melanoma. J Invest Dermatol 74: 379-381
Pack GT, Scharnagel IM (1951) The prognosis for malignant melanoma in the pregnant woman. Cancer 4: 324-334
Pennington DG (1983) Multiple primary melanoma in pregnancy: A case report. Br J Plast Surg 36: 260-261
Rampen FHJ, Mulder JH (1980) Malignant melanoma: an androgen-dependent tumour? Lancet 1: 562-565
Shaw HM, Milton GW, Farago G, McCarthy WH (1978) Endocrine influences on survival from malignant melanoma. Cancer 42: 669-677
Shiu MH, Schottenfeld D, MacLean B, Fortner JG (1976) Adverse effect of pregnancy on melanoma: a reappraisal. Cancer 37: 181-187
Surveillance, epidemiology, and end results (1981) Incidence and mortality data, 1973-77. NCI, Bethesda, pp 98-100 Monograph 57; DHEW publication no. 81-2330
Sutherland CM, Wittliff JL, Fuchs A, Mabie WE (1983 a) The effect of pregnancy on hormone levels and receptors in malignant melanoma. J Surg Oncol 22: 191-192
Sutherland CM, Loutfi A, Mather FJ, Carter CD, Krementz ET (1983 b) Effect of pregnancy upon malignant melanoma. Surg Gynecol Obstet 157: 443-446
Weiss NS, Flannery JT (1978) The relationship of marital status to survival from melanoma. Cancer 42: 296-298
White LP, Linden G, Breslow L, Harzfeld L (1961) Studies on melanoma: the effect of pregnancy on survival in human melanoma. JAMA 177: 235-238

Current Issues in Melanoma Research: Fluorescent Light

Could Melanoma Be Caused by Fluorescent Light? A Review of Relevant Epidemiology

J. M. Elwood

Department of Community Health, University of Nottingham, Queen's Medical Centre, Nottingham NG7 2UH, United Kingdom

Epidemiological Evidence

The first, and at the time of writing still the most substantial, empiric evidence of an association between exposure to fluorescent light and malignant melanoma comes from the study by Beral et al. published in August 1982. The primary aim of this study was to investigate the role of oral contraceptives, so it was restricted to women aged 18-54, and results have been published on this, on pigmentation characteristics and naevi, and on different aspects of sun exposure (Beral et al. 1983, 1984, 1985). This is a retrospective case-control study. Such studies have often given the first evidence of a previously unrecognised cancer causing agent or risk factor, because they can be performed within reasonable lengths of time and require moderate numbers of subjects rather than the huge numbers needed for prospective studies of rare diseases like melanoma. Case-contol studies gave the first good evidence for many important relationships, such as the links between smoking and lung cancer, late age at first birth and breast cancer, sexual activity and uterine cervical cancer, and estrogens and endometrial cancer. The study design is however a complex one which can rarely if ever satisfy all the criteria needed to make the results unambiguous, and has shown some associations which now appear to be spurious, such as that between breast cancer and the use of reserpine.

The case-control study rests on three basic assumptions: that the group of patients with the disease under study is representative of all such patients in terms of the past history of the exposure to the putative causal factor; that the control group chosen gives a group whose exposure to the factor is representative of unaffected subjects; and that the method used to assess past exposure gives sufficiently accurate results and is unbiased. That is to say, the errors in assessment of exposure to the putative causal factor are similar in cases and in controls. If those criteria are met, the measure of association between the causal factor and the disease given by a case-control study will be a valid estimate of the true association, and can be regared in the same way as a result from a prospective cohort study. The association is not necessarily causal, but the causal hypotheses must be assessed against noncausal hypotheses, as discussed below.

Beral et al.'s case series consisted of 287 women aged 15-54 with histologically confirmed melanoma. A later paper shows that 196 had superfical spreading, 42 nodular, and only 4 had lentigo maligna melanoma (Beral et al. 1984). Ideally, the case series should be composed of all newly incident cases from a defined population. These patients were attending the melanoma clinic at Sydney Hospital, but no information on their place of resi-

Recent Results in Cancer Research. Vol 102

dence is given. There were two subseries: 74 "new" cases, newly diagnosed and treated in the clinic between June 1978 (when the study started) and December 1980, all of whom were apparently interviewed, and 213 "old cases" drawn from the 300 "most recently diagnosed" patients seen at the same clinic between 1974 and 1978 (Beral et al. 1984), of whom 213 (71%) were interviewed, the exclusions being due to death (40), illness (3), no trace (16), patient refusal (4), patient living in a remote area (16), and other reasons (8).

Thus, the case series may include patients who came from long distances specifically to this clinic, and excludes a group of patients who had died since diagnosis and a group living in remote areas. The patient group might be expected to be atypical in terms of socioeconomic features, place of residence and perhaps type or degree of spread of melanoma: however, there is nothing to indicate that these limitations would be other than minor. Is it likely that the exposure of these melanoma patients to fluorescent light is similar to that of all melanoma patients from the same source population? The answer is probably yes, so the case series appears acceptable.

The choice of a control series is always difficult and the ideal - subjects truly representative of the unaffected population, except for matching factors, yet assessed under the same conditions as the case series - has perhaps never been obtained. Here, for the new series of 74 cases, 148 hospital inpatients with a range of nonskin conditions were used. Are such subjects likely to have exposures to fluorescent light which are typical of the (undefined) population from which they are drawn? There is no apparent reason why they should not, but as we know little of the epidemiology of fluorescent light exposure, little can be assured. For each of the "old" cases two population controls were used, these being the first women identified as living near to the home of the case patients (presumably the current home, not necessarily that at the time of diagnosis) according to a preset household selection system, more details of which are given in a supplementary letter (Beral and Evans 1982). The system was pursued until two age-matched controls had been successfully interviewed for each case. No information on response rate for the controls is given. Thus, the study has the advantage of having two differently defined control groups, hospital and population based, and a similarity in the results for fluorescent light exposure in the two sets would be encouraging. We are told that "the findings were similar for old and new cases, so the data for the two groups were combined", but the relevant data are not presented.

The third criterion is that the assessment of past exposure to fluorescent light be valid. Let us accept that it must be grossly inaccurate. To obtain an accurate history of such exposure by one interview dealing with events up to 40 years ago is inconceivable. But the history given and the reality might be expected to be reasonably correlated, if adequate recall were encouraged. Details were obtained as part of an occupational history, which covered details of all jobs held for a year or more, and this seems suitable. Given a measure of inaccuracy, did the cases over report their fluorescent light exposure compared to the controls? It can be argued that no specific cause of such a bias is apparent; a causative role of fluorescent light had not been suggested or implied to any of these subjects, as far as we know, and the study dealt primarily with oral contraceptives. As the subjects were more likely to be aware of the postulated links between melanoma and sun exposure, one might expect a stronger bias toward over-reporting of outdoor work. This does not appear to have occurred.

On the other hand, patients with melanoma would be expected to be more interested in any question on a possible causative factor than would patients with no serious disease or a range of unrelated conditions, and for this reason bias, in either direction, cannot be excluded. The more difficult the questions asked, the greater is this possibility, and this may

Table 1. Main results from the study by Beral et al. (1982), giving the number of years of occupational fluorescent light exposure in the 253 women aged 18-54 with melanoma and the 504 age-matched control women, who had always worked indoors

Years of exposure	Melanoma patients *n*	Comparison subjects *n*	Relative risk (RR) and 95% confidence limits
None	25	94	1.0 (reference)
1-9	134	269	1.9 (1.2-3.0)
10-19	80	121	2.5 (1.5-4.2)
20+	14	20	2.6 (1.2-5.9)

Relative risk is the risk or incidence of melanoma in subjects with the given number of years exposure compared with the risk in those with no exposure, who have a reference risk of 1.0
Statistical analysis for trend in the RR from 0 to 20+ years' exposure yields $X^2=9.5$, 1 *d.f.*, $P=0.002$

possibly explain the lack of difference in terms of outdoor exposure. Brown (1982) makes much of the fact that the fluorescent light questions may have acted as a memory trigger, but overstates the case: the questions do not seem too out of place with other details of jobs, such as outdoor work. Such bias would be a greater worry in subsequent retrospective studies, after the publicity given to these initial findings.

So to the results: similarly low proportions of patients and controls had not worked outdoors or had worked partially or totally outdoors, and within the groups whose jobs had been totally indoors, patients reported more years with fluorescent light exposure, the trend being statistically significant, with a two-sided *P* value of 0.002, and being seen both in office workers and in other indoor workers (Table 1).

Confounding was dealt with by presenting the odds ratios and confidence limits for fluorescent light exposure in subsets of each of several potential confounding factors: birthplace (Australia, elsewhere), time spent outdoors in childhood (much, little), main outdoor activity at age 20 (sunbathing, other), frequency of naevi (more than average, average or fewer) and hair colour in childhood (red, blonde, brown or black). Elevated risks were seen in all subgroups except that of subjects with red hair in childhood, although of course several were not statistically significant because of the limited numbers of subjects in each subcategory. These analyses provide some protection against the association being due to confounding by the factors given, but obviously are rather crude. The possibility still remains of confounding, which would be revealed by data on quantitative measures of different types of sun exposure, for example.

Several other points in the data are worthy of note. The data show that the risks were lower in women who were born in Australia, who spent more time outdoors in childhood, or whose main outdoor activity at age 20 was sunbathing; thus, the risk with fluorescent light seems lower if sun exposure is greater, perhaps because of tanning and skin thickening. On the other hand, the risk was higher in women with more naevi than average, a feature also related to greater sun exposure (Holman and Armstrong 1984a). Information on 27 men with melanoma and 35 inpatient controls collected on the basis of the same questionnaire showed a relative risk of 4.4 (95% limits 1.1-17.5) when over 10 or more years of occupational fluorescent light exposure and less than 10 years were compared.

Two items are less consistent. No association was seen with home exposure to fluorescent light, the confidence limits being reasonably narrow (RR=0.9, 95% confidence limits 0.6-1.6). Perhaps the amount of exposure was small, but no information is given. The site distribution showed that those exposed to fluorescent light had an excess of trunk lesions, and no excess on the head and neck or upper limbs. Possibly the usual sun exposure of the head and neck and limbs might make those sites more resistant to fluorescent irradiation, although it is hard to imagine this effect reversing the considerably greater exposure of these sites, both from being uncovered and from being nearer the fluorescent light source in seated office workers. One might expect similar sun exposure of the upper and lower limbs in young female office workers, but much greater exposure of the upper limbs to fluorescent light, giving a relative increase in upper limb tumours.

The interpretation of an association seen in an epidemiological study can be approached in two phases. First, an observed association must be due to one or more of four relationships: causation, bias in the information collected, confounding by one or more factors, or chance variation. Taking the key result of Beral et al. (1982) Table 1, the probability of this result being solely due to chance is about 0.002, given by conventional statistics. This, however, takes no account of the fact that the observation does not result from a study set up to test the hypothesis, but arises as one of presumably many factors assessed in a study designed to look primarily at other issues. How this should affect the assessment of the significance of the finding is not universally agreed. For example, Cole (1979) has argued that it should make little difference, while others have stressed the likelihood of associations arising after examining many variables (Mantel and Haenszel 1959). The issues of confounding and information bias have been discussed above: while there is no particular indication of such influences, they remain as alternative hypotheses.

Secondly, both within this one study and more generally, one can apply the positive criteria which should be fulfilled if a causal relationship exists: such criteria, listed by Hill (1965) and other authorities (U.S. Department of Health, Education and Welfare 1964), generally include the strength of the association, a dose-response relationship, an appropriate time relationship, coherence, plausibility, specificity, reproducibility and experimental verification. Only the time relationship - that cause must precede effect - is absolute.

Of the criteria, the one most clearly shown by the study of Beral et al. (1982) is a dose-response relationship. A regular trend of increasing relative risk with increasing duration of exposure, from never, through, 1-9 and 10-19 to 20+ years, is seen in all indoor workers, in office workers, and to a reasonable extent in other indoor workers (Table 1). Such a relationship is consistent with causation, and is unlikely to occur through biased reporting, but could result from a confounding influence associated quantitatively with duration of exposure to fluorescent lighting. The strength of the association - relative risk around 2.5 for over 10 years' exposure - is only moderate, providing little protection against confounding or bias; but it can be argued that even a strong true effect would not produce a high observed RR, because of the high degree of random error in the assessment of fluorescent light exposure. No information is given about the timing of the exposure; those with more years of exposure presumably had their first exposure earlier, and it is unlikely that enough subjects would have had such discrete and varied timing of exposure as to allow the examination of effects of time since first exposure or age at first exposure. In terms of coherence, Beral et al. point out that the association is consistent with the rapid rise in incidence of melanoma in most populations over the last 30 years and with the higher rates in upper socioeconomic classes and in indoor workers (Lee 1982); also, the association primarily with trunk lesions and least with head and neck lesions fits in with the sites at which incidence has increased most. As to plausibility, this is more difficult and hinges mainly on a consideration of the radiation emissions from fluorescent light and on the role of ultraviolet radiation in the genesis of human malignant melanoma.

Information on the emission spectra of fluorescent lamps is reviewed in the companion paper (Maxwell and Elwood, this volume), which shows that the emissions in the shorter wavelength part of the UVB range (290-295 nm) are sufficiently great in comparison with sunlight to make a causal role plausible if emissions in this range have a specific role in the production of melanoma. While the action spectra for DNA damage, human skin erythema, and the production of nonmelanomatous skin tumours in laboratory animals are similar and show that UVB and shorter wavelengths are the most damaging, the genesis of human melanoma is much less well understood, largely for lack of an animal model. The possible roles of UV in human malignant melanoma have recently been reviewed (Elwood 1984; National Research Council 1982). If it is assumed that the action spectra for the other effects noted above apply to melanoma, a causal role for fluorescent light does seem plausible. At this early stage, little can be said about specificity or, most importantly, reproducibility, which is what the argument must depend on. Experimental verification in human melanoma is not feasible or ethical.

Further Studies of the Fluorescent Light Hypothesis

Five further studies of the hypothesis have been identified, only two of which have been published at the present time of writing; permission to comment on the others has been given by the investigators. These are summarised in Table 2.

Pasternack et al. (1983) briefly reported a study in a letter to the Lancet. They compared 136 melanoma patients from a New York hospital with 282 controls who were patients from the skin clinic without malignant neoplasms. The response rates are not described, nor were the methods of assessment. They found a relative risk of 1.9 (95% confidence limits 1.2, 2.9) with exposure of 35 h or more per week, compared with none from either occupational or home fluorescent lighting in the 5 years before diagnosis; no association was seen with exposures 5-10 years or 10-20 years prior to diagnosis. Thus, these results give some confirmation to the observations of Beral et al.

The other studies reported are essentially negative. Rigel et al. (1983a, b) assessed 114 patients from a different New York hospital, who represented only 30% of the total available patients, and compared them with 228 controls, who comprised staff and patients of the skin and cancer units and had no history of skin cancer. No information is given on the methods of assessment of fluorescent light exposure. No significant difference was seen in terms of average exposure in hours per day. Both these studies are difficult to interpret, because the patients studied represent either a small or an unknown proportion of those available at the centres chosen, the relevance of the control groups chosen is problematical, and the methods of assessment of fluorescent light exposure are not described, making it impossible to assess whether there was adequate protection against biased responses.

Sorahan and Grimley (1985) in Birmingham, England, assessed 58 patients, being 64% of those identified at two hospitals in the city, and two sets of controls, 182 hospital patients and 151 subjects randomly chosen from the Electoral Register. Results were assessed in terms of years of occupational exposure and no significant association was seen. Compared with those with no exposure, the relative risks were 1.2 for 1-9 years' exposure, and 1.7 for 10-19 years' exposure, but then fell to 0.5 for 10 or more years' exposure, producing no overall trend. The recorded risks in relation to fluorescent lights which were on intermittently were higher rather than lower than those related to continuous illumination.

Table 2. Details of five studies set up to examine the possibility of a link between fluorescent lighting and melanoma

Authors	Case series					Control series	Results			Association	Measure used
	Place	Source	Restrictions	Number	Response rate	Source and definition	Number	Response rate	Method of assessment		
Beral et al. (1982)	Sydney, NSW, Australia	One major hospital	a) Women, age 18-54	287	77%	1. Inpatients, excluding chronic, vascular, gynae cologicale gallbladder, breast and mental disease, diabetes, rheumatoid arthritis	148	Unknown	Home or hospital interview	Positive Office stronger None	1. Years of occupational exposure 2. Office or other indoor worker 3. Home exposure
						2. Household sample, matched for age, area of residence	426	Unknown			
			b) Men, age 18-56	27	Unknown	Male inpatients	35	Unknown		Positive	1. Years of occupational exposure
Pasternack et al. (1983)	New York USA	One hospital.	None	136	Unknown	Skin clinic, no neoplasm	282	Unknown	Unknown	Positive Positive None	1. Av. hours/day in previous 5 years 2. Exposure to >35 hours/week 3. Av. hours/day 5-10 years, 10-20 years previously
Rigel et al. (1883a, b)	New York USA	One hospital	None	114	30%	Patients and staff of skin clinic, no neoplasms	228	Unknown	Unknown	None	1. Av. hours/day
Sorahan and Grimley (1985)	Birmingham UK	Two hospitals	Age 20-70	58	64%	1. Random sample from electoral register	151	60%	Postal questionnaire	None	1. Years of occupational exposure
						2. Random sample from hospital discharges excluding skin and mental disease, pregnancy, senility	182	60%			

Elwood et al. (1985)	Nottingham UK	Nottingham residents.	Age 20+	83	74%	In- or outpatients, Nottingham residents	83	92%	Home interview, and postal questionnaire.	None	1. Total hours occupational exposure
										Undiffused stronger	2. Undiffused, diffused and total exposure
										None	3. Home fluorescent light
										Positive	4. Other occupational lighting
English et al. (1985)	Perth, W. Australia	Perth residents	Age 18+	337	68%	Random sample from electoral register	349	63%	Telephone interview following letter	None	1. Years of occupational exposure
										None	2. Total hours and hours/year, home or occupation
										None	3. Total and undiffused exposure
										None	4. Type of room
										None	5. Subtype and subtype analysis

In Nottingham, England, the current author and colleagues (Elwood et al. 1985) assessed 83 melanoma patients, being 74% of all Nottingham residents diagnosed with melanoma in a given period, and compared these with patients chosen from all hospital in- or outpatients during the period. A home interview method was used, and results assessed in terms of total occupational exposure, exposure from total diffused and undiffused sources, home exposure, and exposure to other types of occupational lighting. No consistent significant association was seen with exposure to fluorescent lighting, although the relative risks at maximum total exposures were higher than those for no exposure, the recorded risks were higher in relationship to exposure to undiffused than to diffused lighting, and the total recorded hours of exposure to undiffused lighting were higher in the patients than the controls. Most of these patients were reassessed with the aid of a postal questionnaire, and this showed less evidence of an effect than did the interviews. The study also reported that more cases than controls had been exposed to occupational lighting sources of various types which might be expected to have an ultraviolet component.

The largest study of the topic comes from English et al., in Perth, Western Australia. This study took the opportunity of building on a large and detailed home interview study of melanoma with population-based controls, which was set up previously to study factors other than fluorescent light, including sunlight, moles and naevi, and oral contraceptives (Holman and Armstrong 1984a, b; Holman et al. 1984). After publication of the paper by Beral et al. (1982), these authors went back to the cases and controls interviewed in that study, by sending them a letter with diagrams of various types of lighting fixtures, followed by a telephone interview to record histories of fluorescent lighting exposure. The study is based on 337 residents of Perth who developed melanoma, being 68% of all new cases in the appropriate time period, compared with 349 controls chosen from the electoral rolls and matched for age, sex, and electoral subdivision, representing 91% of the original control group involved in the home interview study, which in turn was 64% of eligible controls. Results are expressed in terms of years of occupational exposure, using an analysis deliberately made analogous to that of Beral et al., and in terms of total exposure and rate of exposure in hours per year from either home or occupational sources, from total and from undiffused sources. Because of the size of the study and the link to the other study, in which cases were carefully clinically and pathologically assessed, results were available by subsites and subtypes of melanoma. In this study, and in the two British studies from Sorahan and Grimley and Elwood et al., possible confounding with measures of outdoor exposure, sun exposure, and host pigmentation factors could also be assessed but did not change the results. The English et al. study shows no association with fluorescent light in terms of all melanomas. There was a significant relationship with unclassified melanoma, with which there are 136 subjects, and a weakly positive trend which was not statistically significant in terms of Hutchison's melanotic freckle (lentigo maligna melanoma) of the head and neck and upper limbs, of whom there were 126. In this study, some information on exposure to other possible ultraviolet sources is given, but no associations were seen, and the number of subjects exposed was small.

Thus the only study supporting the original observations of Beral et al. is that by Pasternack et al. (1983), and for this study at the time of writing we have no information about the methods by which fluorescent light exposure was assessed or on the possible selection effects on either cases or controls. It seems likely that this assessment was done as part of routine clinical work and may well have been different for cases and controls, and the study must be regarded as a weak one. There are now four studies which do not support the original observation and show no consistent and significant association between melanoma and fluorescent light. That of Rigel et al (1983a, b) was beset by the same problems as the study of Pasternack et al. The two British studies of Sorahan and Grimley (1985) and Elwood et al. (1985) have the advantage of assessing melanoma patients appropriately chosen from source populations with known sizes, and use appropriate series of comparison subjects. The study in Nottingham is the only one in which a personal interview system was used, as by Beral et al., and it is interesting that in this study there was more suggestion of a positive relationship with personal interviews than with a subsequent postal questionnaire. This could mean, of course, that the random error is greater in a postal questionnaire survey, but it also raises the possibility that in a direct interview more bias may be introduced. The Birmingham study showed no effect, but the Nottingham study does show trends in the direction of a positive effect, suggesting a possible association with other sources of lighting. The largest study so far available is that of English et al. The case series represents a reasonable proportion of all residents of a given area who had a confirmed diagnosis of melanoma, and the control series is randomly chosen from the source population. The method of assessment, by an initial letter followed by a telephone interview, is relatively fast and simple, and telephone interviews appear to be a useful survey method, (Groves and Kahn 1979); unfortunately no information on the reproducibility of the data obtained, or how it would compare with that collected in a more detailed interview, is available. The results from English et al. are almost totally negative, and in particular there is no indication of a stronger effect of undiffused exposure than of total exposure, stronger effects in relationship to light sources which are likely to be closer, or stronger effects on body sites which are likely to be more directly exposed. The authors point out that there are results which could be interpreted as positive for two subanalyses, that of unclassified melanoma, and of lentigo maligna melanoma of the head and neck and upper limbs, but these represent two of a considerable number of different type- and site-specific analyses, and only the former is statistically significant.

Thus, the available information from other sources does not, on balance, support the original observations of Beral et al. (1982). The most convincing negative result is that of the Western Australia study of English et al. (1985), which in terms of size and sampling methods is comparable to the original study of Beral et al. (1982), while the main suggestion of support for a positive effect comes from the Nottingham study of Elwood et al. (1985), which is the only one to use direct home interviews as used by Beral et al.

Further studies are unlikely to improve on the methods of case and control selection used in the best of the existing studies. However, the results would be more convincing if extensive efforts could be made to take and verify histories of exposure to fluorescent light sources, and this implies an assessment technique, preferably using more than one method of obtaining information, and verification of the answers obtained, for example by talking to those who share the working or the home environment, or by visits to places of employment or to homes to assess the particular types of light fitting. It would also be useful to conduct onsite measurements of ultraviolet emission. Such a study would need to be more ambitious in cost and complexity than those done to date. Prospective designs are virtually impossible in the short term, because of the very large number of subjects needed, as melanoma is still a rare disease even in Australia, and it seems unlikely that a population could be identified in which existing records give information about past fluorescent light exposure. Possibly some very stable occupational groups might be identified.

Thus, the further evaluation of the epidemiological evidence regarding fluorescent light and malignant melanoma needs to wait until case-control studies based on much more detailed methods of assessment become available. The balance of the current epidemiological evidence is that a major causal role of fluorescent light in melanoma remains a possibility but does not seem very likely. However, the potential for health hazards from ultraviolet radiation from fluorescent and from other artificial lighting sources cannot yet be dismissed and requires further work.

References

Beral V, Evans S (1982) Malignant melanoma and exposure to fluorescent lighting at work. Lancet 2: 1227

Beral V, Evans S, Shaw H, Milton G (1982) Malignant melanoma and exposure fluorescent lighting at work. Lancet 2: 290-293

Beral V, Evans S, Shaw H, Milton G (1983) Cutaneous factors related to the risk of malignant melanoma. Br J Dermatol 109: 165-172

Beral V, Evans S, Shaw H, Milton G (1984) Oral contraceptive use and malignant melanoma in Australia. Br J Cancer 50: 681-685

Beral V, Evans S, Shaw H, Milton G (1985) Malignant melanoma, exposure to sunlight and related factors (to be published)

Brown AP (1982) Melanoma and fluorescent light. Lancet 2: 1398

Cole P (1979) The evolving case-control study. J Chron Dis 32: 15-27

Elwood JM (1984) Initiation and promotion actions of ultraviolet radiation on malignant melanoma. In: Borzsonyi M, Day NE, Lapis K, Yamasaki H (eds) Models, mechanisms and etiology of tumour promotion. IARC, Lyon

Elwood JM, Williamson C, Stapleton P (1986) Malignant melanoma in relation to moles, pigmentation, fluorescent and other lighting sources. Br J Cancer 53

English DR, Rouse TL, Zhong X, Watt JD, Holman CDJ, Heenan PJ, Armstrong BK (1985) Cutaneous malignant melanoma and fluorescent lighting. INCI 74: 1191-1197

Groves RM, Kahn RL (1979) Surveys by telephone: a national comparison with personal interviews. Academic, New York

Hill AB (1965) The environment and disease: association or causation? Proc Soc Med 58: 295-300

Holman CDJ, Armstrong BK (1984) Pigmentary traits, ethnic origin, benign nevi, and family history as risk factors for cutaneous malignant melanoma. INCI 72: 257-266

Holman CDJ, Armstrong BK (1984b) Cutaneous malignant melanoma and indicators of total accumulated exposure to the sun: an analysis separating histogenetic types. INCI 73: 75-82

Holman CDJ, Armstrong BK, Heenan PJ (1984) Cutaneous malignant melanoma in women: exogenous sex hormones and reproductive factors. Br J Cancer 50: 673-680

Lee JAH (1982) Melanoma and exposure to sunlight. Epidemiol Rev 4: 110-136

Mantel N, Haenszel W (1959) Statistical aspects of the analysis of data from retrospective studies of disease. J Natl Cancer Inst 22: 719-748

National Research Council (1982) Causes and effects of stratospheric ozone reduction: an update. National Academy Press, Washington DC

Pasternack B, Dubin N, Moseson M (1983) Malignant melanoma and exposure to fluorescent lighting at work. Lancet 1: 704

Rigel DS, Friedman RJ, Levenstein MJ, Greenwald DI (1983a) Malignant melanoma and exposure to fluorescent lighting at work. Lancet 1: 704

Rigel DS, Friedman RJ, Levenstein MJ, Greenwald DI (1983b) Relationship of fluorescent lights to malignant melanoma: another view. J Dermatol Surg Oncol 9: 836-838

Sorahan T, Grimley RP (1985) The aetiological significance of sunlight and fluorescent lighting in malignant melanoma: a case-control study. Br J Cancer 52: 765-769

United States Department of Health, Education and Welfare (1964) Smoking and health: a report of the Advisory Committee to the Surgeon General. DHSS, Washington, DC (PHS publication no. 1103)

Could Melanoma Be Caused by Fluorescent Light? A Review of Relevant Physics

K. J. Maxwell and J. M. Elwood

Department of Physics, University of Nottingham, Queen's Medical Center, Nottingham NG7 2UH, United Kingdom

Fluorescent Lamps

The widespread use of fluorescent lighting dates from the late 1940s. Previously the major source of artificial light was the tungsten filament lamp, which is of relatively low efficiency as most of the radiation it emits is outside the visible range in the infrared (long wavelength) region of the eletromagnetic spectrum and is perceived only by the heat which it produces. The fluorescent tube is a "cold" light source and can be made to produce most of its output in the visible part of the spectrum at wavelengths of 400–700 nm. The luminous efficiency, the amount of useful light output for a given electrical input, can be up to four or five times greater than that of tungsten filament lamps. An added advantage of the fluorescent tube is that it is an extended rather than a point source, and so the light from it has less glare and casts softer shadows.

A fluorescent lamp is essentially a discharge tube in which the discharge is electrically excited in a mercury vapour at low pressure. The radiation from the discharge has relatively little visible component and consists mainly of ultraviolet (UV) radiation of which the dominant wavelength is 254 nm, with subsidiary maxima at 185, 297, 313 and 365 nm, all in the UV region. This UV radiation is absorbed by the powdered phosphor which coats the inner glass surface of the discharge tube and causes the phosphor to emit radiation which is mainly in the visible region of the spectrum. The tube coating thus converts the high-energy short-wavelength radiation produced by the discharge into lower energy visible light (Fig. 1). Ideally, the conversion process produces all its output in the 400- to 700-nm wavelength region, but in practice substantial amounts of higher energy radiation

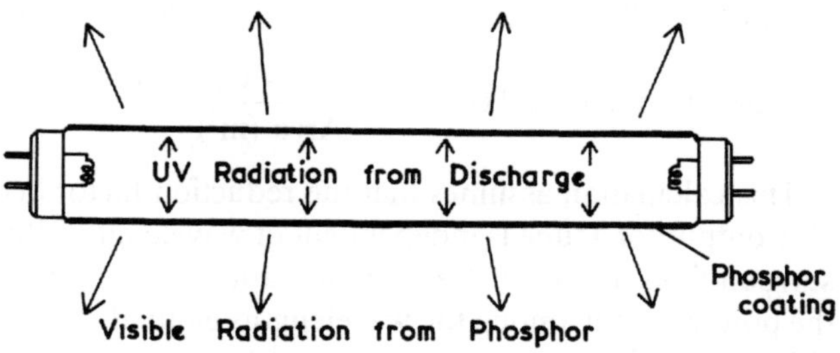

Fig. 1. Fluorescent tube. The electrical discharge produces high-energy UV radiation, which is converted into lower energy visible light by the tube's phosphor coating

at wavelengths below 400 nm remain in the lamp output. At the lower end of the wavelength scale much of this will be absorbed by the glass envelope. In particular, the 254-nm radiation should be totally removed. However, the thin glass may still permit radiation at 290 nm and above to pass through, and the strong 297-nm UV radiation from the mercury discharge will often make some contribution to the lamp's output.

Comparisons of UV Output of Fluorescent Lamps and Sunlight

If we compare the spectrum of a typical fluorescent tube with the spectrum of normal sunlight, then the output of the fluorescent tube will be substantially less than the power of sunlight over most of the optical spectrum. If a causal association between exposure to fluorescent lamps and melanoma exists, we can ask whether there is a region of the UV spectrum where the intensity of radiation from fluorescent tubes may exceed that of the solar intensity at ground level.

Other than a short article by the present authors (Maxwell and Elwood 1983) there appears to be no published quantitative study of this problem. The paper by Rigel et al. (1983) is somewhat less than satisfactory on two counts. First, measurements were carried out only in the range 320–400 nm, i.e., within the so-called UVA band (315–400 nm), and secondly, no attempt was made to look at wavelength bands narrower than the 80-nm resolution of the measuring instrument. There is little doubt, as the trend in the numbers in Tables 1 and 2 will confirm, that the solar irradiance (power per unit area per unit wavelength) is considerably greater than the irradiance from fluorescent tubes at wavelengths of 320 nm and above, and it may be shown that this is true throughout the 320- to 400-nm region with a resolution of 1 nm and for solar elevation down to 10° above the horizon. However, at lower wavelengths in the UVB region (280–315 nm), the comparison between solar irradiance and fluorescent tube irradiance is somewhat different.

The Output of Fluorescent Tubes in the UVB Range (280–315 nm)

The relevant units are:

the LUMEN (lm) (IW at 555 nm = 682 lm for luminous flux
the LUX (illuminance at 1 lm per square metre) for illuminance

However, the rated flux of any tube must be reduced by a utilization factor (UF), which takes into account losses due to geometric factors of the lighting arrangement, factors in the design of light fittings, and the effects of diffusers. A maintenance factor (MF) must be included to allow for the effects of wear on the tube. Thus the relationship becomes: –

$$\text{Average illuminance (lx)} = \frac{\text{Flux (lm)} \times \text{UF} \times \text{MF}}{\text{Area (m}^2\text{)}}$$

This calculation assumes that the reduction factor between actual light output and usable output for a tube is independent of wavelength, although reflections in the fitting and surroundings as well as transmission and scattering by diffusers are likely to redistribute the power output among the wavelengths emitted. No data on such effects is readily available.

Typical values of UF and MF are 0.5 and 0.9, respectively, and typical levels of office illuminance are around 500 lx for general offices and stores and up to 1000 lx for critical drawing tasks and similar work.

Table 1. Spectral power irradiance (μWm^{-2} nm^{-1}) from various fluorescent tubes giving an illuminance of 500 lx

Wavelength (nm)	Tube/Type								
	1	2	3	4	5	6	7	8	9
280	0	0	0	2	0	0	2	0	0
285	0	0	0	2	0	0	2	2	4
290	2	4	4	2	2	2	6	3	4
295	10	53	56	5	3	5	24	16	32
300	17	70	70	8	9	5	37	34	59
305	8	28	25	5	6	13	40	49	71
310	515	865	860	330	319	260	550	613	623
315	413	754	810	280	301	400	560	624	625
320	7	5	4	3	2	490	150	213	238

The table is based on data recorded for 9 of 19 tubes from a leading manufacturer. The other tubes had lower irradiances than those shown

If we assume a level of 500 lx, i.e. 500 lm per m^2, then we may calculate the irradiance in that environment, given that we know the spectral power distribution per unit of luminous flux. This calculation has been carried out for 19 different commonly used tube types produced by a leading manufacturer, and the results for the 9 tubes showing the highest UVB intensities are given in Table 1.

These numbers must now be compared with solar radiation for the various wavelength regions.

Solar Radiation in the UVB Region

Although a substantial amount of the electromagnetic radiation incident on the earth's atmosphere is in the UVB region, ozone in the atmosphere absorbs much of this radiation, resulting in a very rapid decrease in intensity at ground level below 320 nm. The actual cut-off wavelength is the subject of some debate, but most authors agree that it is in the region of 290–295 nm (Fig. 2). This figure depends on such factors as solar altitude, the elevation of the observing site, and the ozone content and the turbidity of the atmosphere. Because of the very high rate of change of intensity of solar radiation with wavelength between 320 nm and 290 nm, these factors are likely to cause very large deviations in the quoted figures for solar irradiance, particularly below 300 nm; a change of 50% in ozone concentration may cause a change of up to a factor of 50 in solar irradiance below 300 nm (Bener 1963). At these wavelengths, much of the measured irradiance may be due not to direct sunlight, but to diffuse Rayleigh scattering of sunlight from the atmosphere. Rayleigh scattering is related to the inverse of the fourth power of wavelength, so that it is stronger for blue light than red and gives the sky its blue colour.

Relevant estimates of solar UV in the appropriate wavelengths are not available. Benér's work, as reviewed in graphical form by Henderson (1977), gives data on wavelengths down to 297.5 nm. Klein and Goldberg (1978) give graphical data on daily average doses for various wavelengths over the year at three different latitudes. These data extend down to 290 nm for the lowest latitude studied, but it is not feasible to work back to the actual spectral power in any wavelength region for a given solar elevation. What can be done is

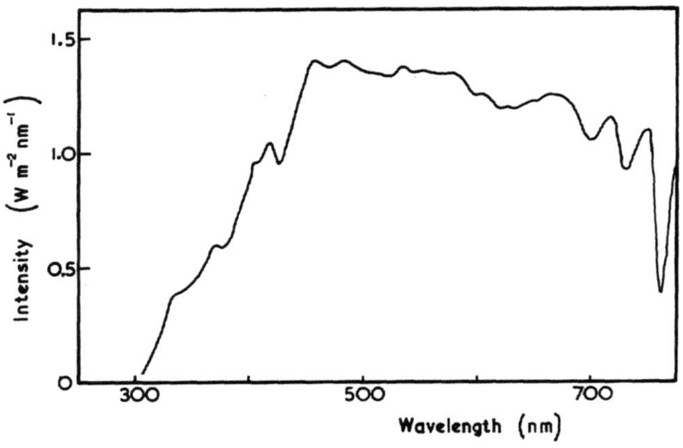

Fig. 2. The spectral distribution of solar irradiance at sea level

Table 2. Solar irradiance at ground level for a 3.3-mm ozone layer ($\mu Wm^{-2} nm^{-1}$)

Wavelength nm	Solar elevation, degrees						
	90	80	70	60	50	40	30
290	0.5	0.4	0.2	0.05	<0.05	–	–
295	160	150	100	50	17	3	0.4
300	5200	4400	3900	2800	1500	600	100

to check the consistency of calculated spectral power figures against this experimental data.

The alternative approach is to use the results of theoretical calculations of solar irradiance at ground level. There are several models to choose from. Robertson (1972) gives figures calculated by Gates (1966), which refer only to direct sunlight and do not include skylight. Green et al. (1974) use a semi-empirical model which calculates the direct and diffuse components separately. For our present purposes, a self-consistent set of numbers for solar spectral power as a function of solar elevation for low wavelengths (less than 320 nm) is required.

The results of Green's equations give numbers which are higher by a factor of two than the measurements of Klein and Goldberg at latitude 39° N and wavelength 295 nm, and higher by a factor of four than those calculated by Gates. However, if Gates' numbers are modified to include the diffuse component and if the departures of the Green model from the measurements of Bener at other wavelengths are considered, then a set of numbers which are in reasonable agreement with the direct measurements of Klein and Goldberg can be produced. The latitude dependence of UVB depends not only on a solar elevation factor, but more strongly on the thickness of the ozone layer, which increases from about 2–2.5 mm at the equator to about 4–4.5 mm near the Poles (Klein and Goldberg 1978). The figures quoted in Table 2 are for an ozone layer of thickness about 3.3 mm, as expected for 30°–40° latitude. There will be small variations of layer thickness during the year. If, indeed, melanoma is UV related, then the variation in its incidence with latitude may be related more to the shift in cut-off wavelength caused by differences in the thicknes of the ozone layer than to differences in solar intensity or duration of exposure.

Comparison of Solar and Fluorescent Light Irradiance

Comparison of Tables 1 and 2 indicates that only below 300 nm is there any direct comparability between the two sources of UVB in terms of irradiance. For wavelengths of 295 nm at the latitude of Sydney, Australia, the spectral power experienced under some fluorescent tubes is comparable to solar spectral power.

In fact, it may be shown that the power of tube 3 exceeds the solar illuminance at all times except when solar elevation exceeds 60°. This condition will occur for about 40% of the year around the summer solstice – for about 3 h either side of noon at the solstice and for about 2 h either side of noon at 1 month from the solstice. The numbers relating to solar irradiance refer chiefly to clear sky conditions, so cloud cover and rain will reduce the solar irradiance below the fluorescent tube irradiance for a substantial number even of the "danger" hours. It is thus reasonable to conclude that in the band around 295 nm, some of the tubes listed in Table 1 will give an irradiance which is comparable to the maximum solar irradiance over most of the year. For lower wavelengths, the flourescent tubes can give irradiances which are an order of magnitude larger than that from the sun at this latitude. This is clearly shown by the 290-nm figures.

The figures in Tables 1 and 2 can be compared in another way. Because of the variability of the sun, both daily and annually, the effective daily "dose rate" at various wavelengths averaged over a 1-year period was calculated. Here, the solar dose at a latitude of 34°, eg., Sydney is taken to be the sum of irradiances throughout the day from sunrise to sunset, taking due account of the variability of the length of day throughout the year and of the variation in solar elevation at different seasons. The fluorescent light dose is taken to be a constant exposure over an 8-h period for 5 days per week and for 50 weeks in the year. In each case, the integrated totals are divided by 365 to give an equivalent average daily dose for easy comparison. The results are presented in Table 3.

These results show that in terms of average UVB dose over an extended period fluorescent tubes give exposures comparable to solar exposure for wavelengths in the region of 295 nm and are an order of magnitude greater at wavelengths around 290 nm. It must further be remembered that by "solar exposure", these results assume unshaded exposure to the sun's rays from sunrise to sunset over the whole year. This is unrealistically high even for outdoor workers, and a truer comparison might result from a reduction in the solar figures; for example, if exposure to sunlight were avoided for a period of about 1 h around midday each day, the solar figures in Table 3 would be reduced by about 20% at 295 nm.

The figures given in Table 1 and Table 3 for fluorescent lighting are also subject to qualification, in that they may be reduced by using diffusers or controllers as part of the light-

Table 3. Comparison of average daily dose of radiation from sunlight and from fluorescent lamps ($\mu J\ cm^{-2}\ mm^{+1}$) between 280 and 300 nm

Wavelength	Solar exposure	Tube type								
		1	2	3	4	5	6	7	8	9
280	0	0	0	0	4	0	0	4	0	0
285	0	0	0	0	4	0	0	4	4	8
290	0.4	4	8	8	4	4	4	12	6	8
295	92	20	106	112	10	6	10	48	32	64
300	471	34	140	140	16	18	10	74	68	118

ing installation. The scale of such reduction depends on light fitting design and on the material from which the diffuser/controller is made. From our personal communications with manufacturers, diffusers giving partial cover only, such as the open lattice type, have very little effect on the UVB content of the resultant illumination. On the other hand, diffusers which completely enclose the tube can have a marked effect on the irradiance figures in the UVB while having very little effect on the overall visible irradiance of the installation. Those diffusers which are manufactured from styrene are claimed to totally remove the UVB content. Those made from acrylic are claimed to remove only 27% of the UVB content. No details on how the figure is distributed over the UVB range at higher resolution are presently available. Thus, it appears that the universal adoption of full-cover styrene diffusers would remove any of the possible melanoma risk suggested by Beral et al.'s (1982) study. As styrene diffusers are generally cheaper than their acrylic counterparts, there is also an economic incentive to switch to styrene.

Conclusions

These results show that in the range of 290–295 nm the intensity of radiation from fluorescent tubes may exceed that of the solar intensity at ground level. The calculations have been carried out for the latitude of 30°.

Is it feasible that the low intensities such as are given out by fluorescent tubes or solar light in the 290- to 295-nm region could be a causal factor for melanoma, even though the intensities at 300 nm and above are very much greater? The mechanism of any skin response producing melanoma is unknown, but it is likely to have an energy threshold. The threshold nature of skin response is exhibited by the erythemal response, which has an energy threshold at a wavelength of about 320 nm. At lower wavelengths, that is higher energy, there is a very rapid increase in erythemal response. It is not the intensity of the radiation which determines the onset of the response, but the energy of the light. Light is made up of "photons" whose energy is given by

$$E = hf = \frac{hc}{\lambda} \quad (1)$$

where λ is wavelength, f is frequency and h and c are constants.

If light does produce a damaging effect at a certain threshold energy, then no matter how large the light intensity may be, that effect will not be induced unless E exceeds the energy threshold, that is unless λ is sufficiently small.

There is a well-known effect shown by many solids which demonstrates this principle – the photoelectric effect. This occurs when light is incident on the surface of a solid and causes an electron to be ejected from the surface. This only occurs above a threshold frequency (f_o) or equivalently below a threshold wavelength (λo), no matter how intense the beam. This threshold is a property, the "work function", of the solid considered. Once the energy of the light photons exceeds the work function of the solid, electrons are ejected with a kinetic energy which depends on the excess energy of the photons over the work function energy,

$$hf = hf_o + \tfrac{1}{2} mv_m^2$$

where v_m is the maximum kinetic energy of electrons mass m liberated by light of frequency f and the work function equals hf_o. The intensity of the light beam becomes important only above the threshold frequency (or below the threshold wavelength). Intensity gives the number of photons in the beam, so determining the number of electrons ejected. Materials showing the effect are generally metals where the electrons are loosely bound.

Skin cells would not be expected to behave in the same way as metals, but it is a general principle of molecular systems that their interaction with light is governed by a quantum photon model, i.e., energy will be transferred from the incident light beam to the receiving material in finite packages or quanta. From Eq. (1) it can be seen that the lower the wavelength of the light, the higher the energy per package. Thus the idea of a threshold wavelength for cell damage in skin is consistent with this model.

The chief issues relevant to any discussion on a relationship between fluorescent light and malignant melanoma are epidemiological and are reviewed in the companion paper (Elwood, this volume). Consideration of the emission spectra of some commonly used fluorescent tubes shows that a causal relationship is plausible if radiation in the 280- to 290-nm region has a role in the development of malignant melanoma. Direct assessment of this by animal experiments is not possible, as an adequate animal model for the production of melanoma by UV radiation does not exist (Elwood 1984), but other biological experimental work may be helpful. Finally, if these studies indicate a connection between melanoma and UVB light, other light sources should be considered which might produce substantial radiation in the same spectral region. This may include lamps found in large cinema projectors, sun lamps, photocopiers, card-readers, and welding equipment and floodlighting equipment using mercury rather than sodium discharges.

References

Bener P (1963) The diurnal and annual variations of the spectral intensity of ultraviolet sky and global radiation at Davos. (Contract AF 61 (052) - 618). Cited in Henderson (1977)

Beral V, Evans S, Shaw H, Milton G (1982) Malignant melanoma and exposure to fluorescent lighting at work. Lancet 2: 290-293

Elwood JM (1984) Initiation and promotion actions of ultraviolet radiation on malignant melanoma. In: Borzsonyi M, Day NE, Lapis K, Yamasaki H (eds) Models, mechanisms and etiology of tumour promotion. IARC, Lyon

Gates DM (1966) Spectral distribution of solar radiation at the earth's surface. Science 151: 523-529

Green AES, Sawada T, Shettle EP (1974) The middle ultraviolet reaching the ground. Photochem Photobiol 19: 251-259

Henderson ST (1977) Daylight and its spectrum. Hilger, London

Klein WH, Goldberg B (1978) Monitoring UVB spectral irradiances at three latitudes. In: Winter FD (ed) Proceedings of the 7th International Solar Energy Conference, New Delhi 1978. Pergamon, New York, pp 400-414

Maxwell KJ, Elwood JM (1983) UV radiation from fluorescent lights. Lancet 2: 579

Rigel DS, Friedman RJ, Levenstein MJ, Greenwald DI (1983) Malignant melanoma and exposure to fluorescent lighting at work. Lancet 1: 704

Robertson DF (1972) Solar ultraviolet radiation in relation to human sunburn and skin cancer. PhD thesis, University of Queensland

Dysplastic Nevus Syndrome and Familial Melanoma

Genetic Aspects of Cutaneous Malignant Melanoma*

M. H. Greene and S. J. Bale

National Cancer Institute, Landow Building, Room 3C29, 7910 Woodmont Avenue, Bethesda, MD 20892, USA

Historical Perspective

For those of us engaged in studying familial cancer in general, and familial melanoma in particular, it is both fitting and fascinating to learn that the first patient with malignant melanoma of the skin described in the English language literature was a member of a melanoma-prone family (Norris 1820). Writing in 1820, describing a patient he had treated 3 years earlier, Dr. William Norris (an eminent Scottish surgeon of the day) reported in graphic detail the now all-too-familiar downhill course of far-advanced, widely disseminated melanoma. At the end of his vivid clinical case report, Norris noted "It is remarkable that this gentleman's father, about thirty years ago, died of a similar disease .... This tumor originated in a mole, and it will be worth mentioning that not only my patient and his children had many moles on various parts of their bodies, but also his own father and brothers had many of them .... These facts, together with a case that has come under my notice rather similar, would incline me to believe that this disease is hereditary." Thus, Norris both described the first melanoma-prone kindred and raised the hypothesis that its melanoma susceptibility was related to the presence of numerous moles.

This cogent set of clinical observations lay fallow until 1952, at which time Cawley reported on a similar family (Cawley 1952), thus opening the modern era of interest in familial melanoma. Cawley's kindred included a father, son, and daughter with cutaneous malignant melanoma (CMM); like Norris, he commented upon the presence of "numerous nevi" in the two sibs who were affected with CMM (but not in the father). He reviewed the clinical literature, which consisted of several families in which intraocular melanoma had been reported, but found no examples of multiple-case skin melanoma kindreds (he evidently was unaware of Norris' earlier report). He further reviewed the experimental literature, and concluded that various studies of melanoma in fishes, reptiles, rodents, swine, and horses had documented the influence of heredity upon melanoma susceptibility in animals. He felt that the family he described indicated that "heredity, not the other intrinsic or extrinsic factors in the origin of cancer, and not chance, was evidently the noxious agent ...." He acknowledged, appropriately, that one could not prove Mendelian inheritance on the basis of a single family.

Since Cawley's seminal report, numerous families with multiple cases of CMM have been reported. In many of these kindreds the presence of numerous nevi was commented

* *Abbreviations: CMM,* cutaneous malignant melanoma; *DNS,* dysplastic nevus syndrome

Recent Results in Cancer Research. Vol 102

upon, and other characteristics of CMM-prone families emerged. In particular, the unusually young age at CMM diagnosis and the predisposition of such patients for developing multiple independent primary CMM were recognized (Greene and Fraumeni 1979). However, the basis of melanoma susceptibility in these families remained obscure, and the hypothesis that familial CMM represented a true Mendelian trait remained untested. Twin studies, one classic approach to assessing the genetic component of a given disease, have contributed very little to our understanding of melanoma genetics. To our knowledge, this question has never been formally addressed in a twin study. There are, however, occasional case reports of melanoma in twins, the best known of which is that of St.-Arneault et al. (1970), who described the development of CMM in a pair of monzygotic twins. Particular interest attached to the fact that tumor diagnosis was nearly simultaneous in the two patients, and that both melanomas arose at the same location on the skin. While interesting, such observations provide little quantitative proof for a genetic disease mechanism.

A more systematic attempt to address this issue was undertaken by Anderson, who conducted a medical record review of 2164 consecutive melanoma patients treated at the M.D. Anderson Hospital (Anderson 1971). Thirty-six multiplex families were identified; using a procedure which by its dependence upon nonsystematically taken family histories (with no effort made to document reported instances of melanoma in relatives) almost certainly resulted in underascertainment of familial clusters. Anderson observed the differences between familial and nonfamilial CMM patients noted above, and further concluded that the probability of these familial clusters occurring by chance alone was very small. By inspecting the pattern of melanoma distribution in these 36 families, he indicated that the genetics of familial melanoma were likely to entail an autosomal mechanism, but that the mode of inheritance was "complex", perhaps polygenic in nature. Anderson also observed that children of affected females in his sample were more likely to develop melanoma than were the offspring of affected males, and concluded that a maternal cytoplasmic mechanism might be a factor in susceptibility to familial melanoma.

Wallace and colleagues observed 42 multiple-case families among the families of 473 index patients with CMM identified through the Queensland Melanoma Project (Wallace et al. 1973). Without applying quantitative methods, they concluded that there was no pattern which resembled the action of a single gene in these 42 families. They interpreted their data as indicating that there was a real genetic component in the etiology of CMM, but that it was probably polygenic in its basis. In part, this conclusion was based upon an earlier, smaller survey by the same investigators, in which a study of 923 first-degree relatives of 125 consecutive patients with CMM resulted in an estimate of the heritability of liability to melanoma of 11% (Wallace et al. 1971). They acknowledged the difficulty of distinguishing between polygenic inheritance and dominant inheritance with incomplete penetrance, but felt that the increased risk to further relatives observed in families with more than one affected member and the tendency for the probands of families with multiple cases to show more extreme forms of the disease argued in favor of a polygenic mechanism.

Further support for the notion of polygenic inheritance has been provided more recently by Duggleby et al. (1981) in their case-control study of malignant melanoma. They assessed the risk of melanoma in the relatives of cases and controls in their study, and concluded that the presence of an autosomal dominant gene was unlikely. Half the liability to melanoma in their study could be attributed to the additive effect of many genes, each with a small effect. One methodologic point of concern was the manner in which affected family members were ascertained. This study was conducted in western New York State;

affected family members were identified by linking information obtained through interview to data contained in the New York State Tumor Registry. Thus, relatives whose residence was outside the State of New York could not be identified through this procedure. Further, relatives who lived in New York City were also not ascertainable, since New York City does not participate in the New York State Tumor Registry. Thus, the potential for significant underascertainment of family members seems substantial. Some evidence from this study supports such a possibility: only 2% of CMM probands were found to have a positive family history of melanoma, while most previous surveys have suggested that 5%-10% of carefully evaluated melanoma probands will be found to have a positive family history (Greene and Anderson unpublished observation; Greene and Fraumeni 1979).

Contemporary Studies

Recent efforts toward elucidating the genetics of familial melanoma have been influenced by the recognition of the dysplastic nevus syndrome (DNS) (Clark et al. 1978; Greene 1984; Greene et al. 1980; Reimer et al. 1978). In the course of evaluating a series of melanoma-prone families, we noticed that melanoma patients and some of their unaffected blood relatives had very unusual moles (nevi) on their skin. These lesions differed from ordinary common acquired (junctional, compound or dermal) nevi in that they tended to be more numerous, larger than normal, irregularly shaped and variably pigmented, and located at body sites where common nevi only rarely occur (Elder et al. 1982; Reimer et al. 1978). These nevi have both a characteristic clinical (Elder et al. 1982; Greene et al. 1985; Reimer et al. 1978) and a distinctive histological appearance (Clark et al. 1984, 1978; Elder et al. 1981), which makes it possible to identify them as a separate class of melanocytic lesions. It has been well documented that dysplastic nevi are the precursors of most familial melanomas. Within melanoma-prone families, it is now possible to distinguish those specific family members who are at high risk of melanoma (those with either dysplastic nevi or a previous melanoma) from those whose melanoma risk is nearly normal (Greene et al., 1985). It is clear, of course, that some melanoma-prone families do not have the DNS (dysplastic nevus syndrome), but such kindreds seem to be in the minority.

The bulk of these observations were made in the course of studying a series of melanoma-prone kindreds in great detail. We have evaluated 401 members of 14 high-risk families, and conducted a series of clinical, laboratory, and genetic studies designed to clarify the pathogenesis of familial melanoma. With reference to formal genetic analysis, we applied the Elston-Stewart maximum likelihood method of segregation analysis to these 14 high-risk families, after having classified each family member with regard to melanoma status and DNS status. In nearly all cases, the diagnosis of either CMM or DNS was made on both clinical and histological data. When segregation analysis was conducted with only those family members with melanoma considered to be affected, the distribution of cases was compatible with an autosomal dominant mode of inheritance (Greene et al. 1983). Both x-linked and recessive models were clearly ruled out. Since our clinical observations indicated that nearly all the melanomas developing in these family members arose from dysplastic nevi (Greene et al., in press), we conducted a second segregation analysis to determine whether the distribution of these melanoma precursors was also compatible with an autosomal dominant mode of inheritance. In this analysis, family members were considered to be "affected" if they had either CMM or DNS. To our surprise and concern, none of the genetic models tested fit these data well; we could not demonstrate Mendelian inheritance for the combined CMM/DNS phenotype (or, in fact, for DNS alone). A dominant model failed to fit the data because $\tau 2$, the probability that an affected heterozygote transmits the disease to his or her offspring, was estimated to be 1.0 in these families, rather than 0.5 as expected with the assumption of a dominant hypothesis. Thus, there were "too many" family members with DNS. We considered various explanations for this finding. One concern was that we might have overdiagnosed DNS, thus inappropriately classifying some family members as affected when in fact they were not. To test this possibility, we conducted a third analysis in which family members were classified as affected by the DNS only if they had at least two biopsy-proven dysplastic nevi; the result was the same.

While our data probably will never permit a final and definitive resolution of this problem, the most likely explanation is based upon the knowledge that one of the fundamental assumptions of segregation analysis is violated by our data. Implicit in segregation analysis is the assumption that the disease phenotype is rare in genotypically normal individuals. At the outset of our study, we believed that dysplastic nevi were unique precursors to familial melanoma only, and that the aforementioned assumption was correct. It has subsequently become apparent that there is a nonfamilial type of dysplastic nevus and that this entity may be surprisingly common in the general poulation. Histological evidence has revealed the presence of a dysplastic nevus at a margin of one-third to one-half of *all* primary melanomas (Clark et al. 1984; Elder et al. 1981; Rhodes et al. 1983), and clinical evaluation of unselected melanoma patients has shown that a similar proportion have clinical evidence of DNS (Rhodes et al. 1980; Swerdlow et al. 1984; Taylor et al. 1984), even in the absence of a family history of melanoma. More recently, 4.8% of 881 consecutive patients seen in a private dermatology practice for problems unrelated to pigmented skin lesions were shown to have biopsy-proven dysplastic nevi (Crutcher and Sagebiel 1984). Since these nonfamilial dysplastic nevi are (currently) indistinguishable from their familial counterparts by either clinical or microscopic examination, it is possible that some members of our study families have the nonfamilial form of the DNS. Such persons would be phenotypically abnormal/genotypically normal individuals, a phenomenon which could create the distorted segregation ratio noted above. The possibility that such events might have occurred in our study population is supported by the observation that 4 of 91 spouses examined were found to have DNS. This seems to be the best and most likely explanation for our inability to demonstrate that the DNS trait segregates in an autosomal dominant fashion.

An analysis of the segregation of the combined CMM/DNS phenotype in four families by less sophisticated analytic techniques also suggested an autosomal dominant pattern of inheritance (Lynch et al. 1983). Further support for the possibility that DNS is truly a dominant trait was provided by the linkage analysis conducted in our cohort of patients. Linkage analysis of the CMM/DNS phenotype versus a panel of genetically determined polymorphic markers revealed a lod score of 1.56 for the Rhesus blood group locus, at a recombination fraction (θ) of 30% (Greene et al. 1983). This analysis was conducted under the assumption of autosomal dominant inheritance and used the parameter estimates obtained from the melanoma-only segregation analysis. Detection of linkage between the CMM/DNS phenotype and a known genetic marker, under these conditions, provides additional evidence for dominant inheritance. If one were to assume complete penetrance, the maximum lod score between the CMM/DNS trait and the *Rh* locus would be 2.01. It is generally felt that a lod score of $\geqslant 3.0$ is required for proof of linkage; thus, our observations regarding CMM/DNS and the *Rh* locus must be regarded as suggestive and certainly worthy of further investigation, but not definitive. Additional studies are now under way with DNA restriction fragment length polymorphisms as genetic markers, to clarify whether this observation is real. Our data imply that a familial melanoma susceptibility gene may be located near the *Rh* gene, on the short arm of chormosome 1. This hypothesis receives some support from the finding that chromosome 1p is the most frequently abnormal genomic segment in human melanoma tumor cells (Balaban et al. 1984). However, other locations for a melanoma susceptibility gene have been proposed.

To extract the maximum amount of information from the data collected in our 14 family survey, we have applied several additional analytic techniques to the question of what genetic model (if any) best fits the CMM/DNS phenotype (Bale et al. 1985a). One approach has entailed the use of life-table techniques designed to test genetic hypotheses for diseases with a late, variable age of onset (Chase et al. 1983). This technique permits estimation of the probability of disease onset by a given age, using data from persons of all ages in the study. Such a strategy circumvents the cross-sectional nature of our family study data set, at least in part, and should produce a more accurate estimate of the segregation ratio than a simple count of affected persons among all those at risk. Since CMM is a disease of late and variable age at onset, and since DNS is usually manifest by the age of 20, the life-table approach should prove particularly useful in assessing the mode of disease transmission. This technique also allows an analysis of the CMM trait, i.e., ascertainment bias. One could argue that the segregation data described above for CMM alone are distorted owing to our enrollment of multiple-case families in this study. Since the DNS status of study participants was unknown when these families were enrolled in the project, the use of dysplastic nevi to identify probands avoids the bias inherent in using melanoma status for this purpose.

The 14 pedigrees were coded so that the investigator was blind to the melanoma status of all family members. Forty-six probands with DNS were identified, and the risk of melanoma among their relatives was evaluated by Chase's method (Chase et al. 1983). In a similar fashion, a cohort of relatives of melanoma patients was identified, and the risk of DNS was determined. The Kaplan-Meier estimate of the probability of escaping melanoma for the first-degree relatives of the DNS probands was 0.54; thus, the estimated segregation ratio for the CMM trait was 0.46, a value not significantly different from the predicted value of 0.50 for autosomal dominant inheritance. This analysis permits estimation of the penetrance of the melanoma gene: 91%. Similarly, 35 family members with melanoma defined 116 first-degree relatives at risk of DNS. In these data, 54% of person at risk were affected by the DNS. Once again, this value does not differ significantly from the theoretical value of 0.50. Both analyses thus provide further support for an autosomal dominant mode of inheritance for both CMM and DNS (Bale et al. 1985a).

Since there is evidence that both the CMM and the DNS traits are consistent with autosomal dominant inheritance, it is theoretically acceptable to test for linkage between the two loci which control their expression. Why would one wish to do such an analysis? One of the principal hypotheses in our studies of familial melanoma and its precursors is the possibility that the same gene predisposes to both conditions, i.e., that there is pleiotropy of effect for this cancer susceptibility gene. If this hypothesis is correct, one would predict that linkage analysis between the two traits would yield a high lod score (i.e., the "two" genes would be linked) and a recombination fraction of zero (i.e. the "two" genes would be identical). Linkage analysis of the two traits in our cohort of 14 families gave an interpolated maximum lod score of 3.86 at $\theta = 0.08$ (Bale et al. 1985a). This very small recombination fraction is not significantly different from 0; the fact that θ is not equal to 0 is probably accounted for by the fact that these genes are incompletely penetrant (Bale et al. 1985a) submitted; Greene et al. 1983; Lynch et al. 1983). Thus, these analyses imply that

DNS and hereditary melanoma result from the pleiotropic action of a single, highly penetrant gene behaving in an autosomal dominant manner.

As noted earlier, other suggestions have been put forward regarding the genomic location of a melanoma susceptibility gene. The most prominent candidate, aside from chromosome 1p, is chromosome 6p, the location of the human major histocompatibility complex. Several lines of evidence provide reasons to hypothesize that a melanoma susceptibility gene might be linked to HLA in man. First, the *HLA* region is the location of a number of genes which control and regulate immune function, and patients with acquired or genetically determined immunodeficiency conditions are known to be at increased risk of developing melanoma (Greene et al. 1981; Tucker et al. 1985). Furthermore, several groups of investigators have reported the presence of subtle immunologic abnormalities in members of melanoma-prone families (Dean et al. 1979; Hersey et al. 1981; Vandenbark et al. 1979). In addition, the elegant experimental work of Kripke's group has provided a rodent model which offers a nexus between immune function and ultraviolet radiation (the strongest currently accepted risk factor for melanoma, aside from mole number) in the pathogenesis of CMM (Kripke 1984). Population studies comparing the distribution of HLA phenotypes of unrelated melanoma patients and unaffected persons, including at least one very good study (Barger et al. 1982), have identified significant differences between cases and controls at the *HLA-DR* locus. Thus, there is ample reason to explore the relationship between the *HLA* region and the risk of familial melanoma. In family studies, of course, one has the opportunity to assess linkage as well as association, and several reports have suggested that a melanoma susceptibility gene may be linked to HLA. A single family reported from Australia yielded a lod score of 2.0 between the melanoma trait and *HLA* haplotype (Hawkins et al. 1981). The DNS status of this family was not known, and thus the combined CMM/DNS phenotype was not assessed. HLA studies in a series of European families have also been reported, but formal linkage analysis was not performed (Pellegris et al. 1982). These investigators concluded that the melanoma trait was linked to HLA in some families but not in others, based on inspection of the pedigrees.

We have HLA-typed 11 of the 14 families in our cohort study, and have conducted linkage analysis between HLA and the CMM trait as well as the combined CMM/DNS phenotype (Bale et al. 1985b). This analysis has yielded large negative lod scores between HLA and CMM alone (lod $= -68.99$ at $\theta = 0.01$) and CMM/DNS (lod $= -65.56$ at $\theta = 0.01$). In the aggregate, these results provide very strong evidence against linkage between these traits and the *HLA* region in our families. It is noteworthy that one of the 11 families tested did show a lod score of 1.3 (at $\theta = 0.1$) when considered alone, but in the aggregated data set this finding was overwhelmed by the large negative lod scores in other families. Formal testing revealed no evidence for heterogeneity of recombination values either in our data set or within the data set created by pooling our own with previously published data. We did observe heteroeneity *between* our data and those previously published, a finding most probably attributable to investigators' tendency to publish positive findings preferentially.

One might reasonably inquire "How important, in practical terms, is hereditary melanoma?" After all, this must be an incredibly rare condition. In fact, familial aggregations of melanoma occur with surprising frequency. In a survey of 405 consecutive, newly diagnosed CMM patients seen at the M.D. Anderson Hospital in whom a detailed, careful family history was taken and verified, 32 patients (8%) had a *proven* family history of melanoma (Greene and Anderson, unpublished observations). Family history is also a risk factor that is now being assessed in a series of case-control studies of melanoma. Most recently, the Australian study of Holman and Armstrong (1984) has shown that the risk of melanoma increases as a function of the number of relatives reported to have melanoma, with the odds ratio increasing from 2.3 to 5.0 in patients with one and two affected relatives, respectively (both ratios significantly different from 1.0, persons with 0 affected relatives). The use of multivariate techniques for simultaneous assessment of the three strongest melanoma risk factors in this study (number of nevi, cutaneous phenotype, and family history) yielded a relative risk of melanoma in patients with one or more affected blood relatives of 2.4 ($P=0.003$). Thus, it is clear that the familial contribution to melanoma susceptibility is a significant one. Our data derived from melanoma-prone families suggest that this familial risk factor is, in fact, a genetic predisposition to melanoma.

Animal Models of Melanoma

Many investigators have used animal models to study melanoma etiology. Since animals can be bred selectively in controlled environments, they provide research opportunities not available to those of us who study human genetics. A specific mouse strain, C57BL/6, has been used for this purpose (Berkelhammer et al. 1982), as have guinea pigs (Clark et al. 1976) and *Drosophila* (Sang 1969). Certain breeds of horses are well-known for their melanoma susceptibility (Fitzpatrick et al. 1950), and the Sinclair swine has attracted considerable attention recently because it bears melanocytic precursor lesions which some investigators have linkened to dysplastic nevi (Manning et al. 1974). However, unlike dysplastic nevi, the lesions found in Sinclair swine are congenital, rather than acquired.

The animal model which has been most extensively studied, and is currently the best understood, is the occurrence of melanoma in the fish species *Xiphophorus,* most particularly in swordtails and platyfish. This model was developed more than 55 years ago (Gordon 1927; Haussler 1928; Kosswig 1927) and has received considerable attention recently. In brief, all these fishes have a tumor gene, designated *"Tu,"* which has been mapped to the X chromosome. The expression of *Tu* is under the control of several linked and some nonlinked regulatory genes known as *"R"* genes (Anders et al. 1973), the most important of which is the *Esterase-1*-linked gene *"Diff"* (Morizot and Siciliano 1983). When *R-Diff* is in the homozygous state, it leads to suppression of melanoma development in the fish (Ahuja et al. 1980; Scholl 1980; Siciliano and Wright 1976). However, *Tu* can be separated from *R-Diff* and other linked *R* genes by translocation from the X chromosome to another genomic site. When this occurs, *Tu* is free to effect its transforming activities on the melanophore system, resulting in the development of malignant melanoma (Anders and Anders 1978). Mutations or otherwise turning off, of other *R* genes result in variable alterations in the expression of *Tu,* ranging from total-body involvement with malignant melanoma to the development of discrete, isolated colonies of neoplastically transformed melanophores. These data suggest that *Xiphophorus* melanoma is effected by *R* gene dosage, i.e., that neoplasia is a conditional event dependent upon the degree of impairment or deletion of regulatory gene function. Recent evidence has implicated the activity of oncogenes in the pathogenesis of melanoma in *Xiphophorus* (Anders 1982), providing still further avenues of parallel research for human melanoma.

Conclusion

One hundred and sixty-five years ago, an alert clinician recognized the implications of a familial cluster of malignant melanoma of the skin. He observed that the melanoma patients in this family were unusually moley, and speculated that this condition was hereditary. The full import of his insight is only now being realized: the evidence available to date indicate that there is, in fact, a genetic variant of malignant melanoma in man, and that it behaves as an autosomal dominant Mendelian trait. Furthermore, not only are melanoma-prone family members unusually moley; in addition, the moles themselves comprise a unique clinicopathologic entity, a class of melanocytic lesions which are unusually susceptible to malignant transformation. There are now clues to the genomic location of the locus which predisposes to malignant melanoma in families, clues which are being pursued with the very latest techniques of molecular biology. These findings have led to advances in the prevention and detection of melanoma in high-risk families, and raised the likelihood of identifying high-risk individuals in the general community as well. Looking back to the work of Norris, we have made some progress: at a minimum, we could provide him with tools for more effective management of the members of the family he described so vividly. We expect that when our descendants look back on us, 165 years hence, still further progress will have been made. It is entirely possible that melanoma as a disease will exist no longer, its ravages eliminated by the discovery of the gene product which is at the heart of the hereditary form of this condition.

References

Ahuja MR, Schwab M, Anders F (1980) Linkage between a regulatory locus for melanoma cell differentiation and an esterase locus in Xiphophorus. J Heredity 71: 403-407

Anders F (1982) The biology of an oncogene, based upon studies on neoplasia in Xiphophorus. In: Jaenicke L (ed) Biochemistry of differentiation and morphogenesis. Springer, Berlin Heidelberg New York, pp 91-115

Anders F, Anders A (1978) Etiology of cancer as studied in the platyfishswordtail system. Biochem Biphys Acta 516: 61-95

Anders F, Anders A, Klinke K (1973) Regulation of gene expression in the Gordon-Kosswig melanoma system. In: Schroder JH (ed) Genetics and mutagenesis of fish. Springer, Berlin Heidelberg New York, pp 33-52

Anderson DE (1971) Clinical characteristics of the genetic variety of cutaneous melanoma in man. Cancer 28: 721-725

Balaban G, Herlyn M, Guerry D, et al. (1984) Cytogenetics of human malignant melanoma and premalignant lesions. Cancer Genet Cytogenet 11: 429-439

Bale SJ, Chakravarti A, Greene MH (1985a) Cutaneous malignant melanoma and familial dysplastic nevi - evidence for autosomal dominance and pleiotropy. Am J Hum Genet (in press)

Bale SJ, Greene MH, Mann D, Murray C, Goldin L, Johnson AH (1985b) Familial malignant melanoma is not linked to the HLA complex on chromosome 6. Int J Cancer 36: 439-443

Barger BO, Acton RT, Soong S-J, Roseman J, Balch C (1982) Increase in HLA-DR4 in melanoma patients from Alabama. Cancer Res 42: 4276-4279

Berkelhammer J, Oxenhandler RW, Hook RR Jr, Hennessy JM (1982) Development of a new melanoma model in C57BL/6 mice. Cancer Res 42: 3157-3163

Cawley EP (1952) Genetic aspects of malignant melanoma. AMA Arch Dermatol 65: 440-450

Chase GA, Foldstein MF, Breitner JC, Beatty TH, Self SG (1983) The use of life tables and survival analysis in testing genetic hypotheses, with an application to Alzheimer's disease. Am J Epidemiol 117: 590-597

Clark WH Jr, Min BH, Kligman LHL (1976) The developmental biology of induced malignant melanoma in guinea pigs and a comparison with other neoplastic system. Cancer Res 36: 4079-4091

Clark WH Jr, Reimer RR, Greene MH, Ainsworth AM, Mastrangelo MJ (1978) Origin of familial melanoma from heritable melanocytic lesions: the B-K mole syndrome. Arch Dermatol 114: 732-738

Clark WH Jr, Elder DE, Guerry D, Epstein MN, Greene MH, Van Horn M (1984) A study of tumor progression: the precursor lesions of superficial spreading and nodular melanoma. Hum Pathol 15: 1147-1165

Crutcher WA, Sagebiel RW (1984) Prevalence of dysplastic naevi in a community practice. Lancet 1: 729

Dean J, Greene MH, Reimer RR, LeSane FV, McKeen EA, Mulvihill JJ, Blattner WA, Herberman RB, Fraumeni JF Jr (1979) Immunologic abnormalities in melanoma-prone families. JNCI 63: 1139-1145

Duggleby WF, Stoll H, Priore HL, Greenwald P, Graham S (1981) A genetic analysis of melanoma-polygenic inheritance as a threshold trait. Am J Epidemiol 114: 63-72

Elder DE, Greene MH, Bondi EE, Clark WH Jr (1981) Acquired melanocytic nevi and melanoma - the dysplastic nevus syndrome. In: Ackerman AB (ed) Pathology of malignant melanoma. Masson, New York, pp 185-215

Elder DE, Greene MH, Guerry D, Kraemer KH, Clark WH Jr (1982) The dysplastic nevus syndrome: our definition. Am J Dermatopathol 4: 445-460

Fitzpatrick TB, Lerner AB, Calkins E, Summerson WH (1950) Malignant melanoma in horses. Proc Soc ExBiol Med 75: 394-410

Gordon M (1927) The genetics of a viviparous top-minnow platypoecilus; the inheritance of two kinds of melanophores. Genetics 12: 253-283

Greene MH (1984) The dysplastic nevus syndrome. Hosp Pract 19: 91-108

Greene MH, Fraumeni JF Jr (1979) The hereditary variant of malignant malanoma. In: Clark WH Jr, Goldman LI, Mastrangelo MJ (eds) Human malignant melanoma. Grune and Stratton, pp 139-166

Greene MH, Clark WH Jr, Tucker MA, Elder DE, Kraemer KH, Fraser MC, Bondi EE, Guerry D, Tuthill R, Hamilton R, LaRossa D (1980) Precursor nevi in cutaneous malignant melanoma - a proposed nomenclature. Lancet 2: 104

Greene MH, Young TI, Clark WH Jr (1981) Malignant melanoma in renal transplant recipients. Lancet 1: 1196-1199

Greene MH, Goldin LR, Clark WH Jr, Lourien E, Kraemer KH, Tucker MA, Elder DE, Fraser MC, Rowe S (1983) Familial malignant melanoma: autosomal dominant trait possibly linked to the Rh locus. Proc Natl Acad Sci USA 80: 6071-6075

Greene MH, Clark WH Jr, Tucker MA, Elder DE, Kraemer KH, Guerry D, Witmer WK, Thompson J, Matozzo I, Fraser MC (1985) Acquired precursors of cutaneous malignant melanoma - the familial dysplastic nevus syndrome. N Engl J Med 312: 91-97

Greene MH, Clark WH Jr, Tucker MA, et al. (1985) The high risk of malignant melanoma in melanoma-prone families with dysplastic nevi. Ann Intern Med 102: 458-464

Haussler G (1928) Über Melanombildung bei Bastarden von Xiphophorous helleri und Platypoecilus maculatus var. rubra. Klin Wochenschr 7: 1561-1562

Hawkins BR, Dawkins RL, Hockey A, Houliston JB, Kirk RL (1981) Evidence for linkage between HLA and malignant melanoma. Tissue Antigens 17: 540-541

Hersey P, Edwards A, Honeyman M, McCarthy WH (1981) Low natural killer cell activity in familial melanoma patients and their relatives. Br J Cancer 40: 113-122

Holman CD, Armstrong BK (1984) Pigmentary traits, ethnic origin, benign nevi and family history as risk factors for cutaneous malignant melanoma. JNCI 72: 257-266

Kosswig C (1927) Über Bastarde der teleostier Platypoecilus und Xiphophorus. Ztschrift für induktive Abstammungs und Vererbungslehre 44: 253

Kripke ML (1984) Immunological unresponsiveness induced by ultraviolet radiation. Immunol Rev 80: 87-102

Lynch HT, Fusaro RM, Kimberling WJ, Lynch JF, Shannon Danes B (1983) Familial atypical multiple mole-melanoma (FAMMM) syndrome-segregation analysis. J Med Genet 20: 342-344

Manning PJ, Milliken LE, Cox VS, Carey KD, Hook RR Jr (1974) Congenital cutaneous and visceral melanomas of Sinclair miniature swine: three case reports. JNCI 52: 1559-1566

Morizot D, Siciliano M (1983) Linkage group V of platyfishes and swordtails of the genus Xiphophorus: linkage of loci for malate dehydrogenase-2, esterase-1 and esterase-4 with a gene controlling the severity of hybrid melanoma. JNCI 71: 809-813

Norris W (1820) A case of fungoid disease. Edinb Med Surg J 16: 562-565

Pellegris G, Illeni MT, Rovini D, Vaglini M, Cascinelli N, Ghidoni A (1982) HLA complex and familial malignant melanoma. Int J Cancer 29: 621-623

Reimer RR, Clark WH Jr, Greene MH, Ainsworth A, Fraumeni JF Jr (1978) Precursor lesions in familial melanoma. A new genetic preneoplastic syndrome. JAMA 239: 744-746

Rhodes AR, Sober AJ, Mihm MC Jr, Fitzpatrick TB (1980) Possible risk factors for primary cutaneous melanoma. Clin Res 28: 252A

Rhodes AR, Harrist TJ, Day CL, Mihm MC Jr, Fitzpatrick TB, Sober AJ (1983) Dysplastic melanocytic nevi in histologic association with 234 primary cutaneous melanomas. J Am Acad Dermatol 9: 563-574

St.-Areault G, Nagel G, Kirkpatrick D, Kirkpatrick R, Holland JF (1970) Cutaneous malignant melanoma in identical twins from a set of triplets. Cancer 25: 672-677

Sang JH (1969) Biochemical basis of hereditary melanotic tumors in *Drosophila*. NCIM 31: 291-301

Scholl E (1980) Untersuchungen über biochemische Marker bei verschiedenen Genotypen lebendgebärender Zahnkarpten der Gutlung *Xiphophorus*. Doctoral dissertation, University of Giessen

Siciliano MJ, Wright DA (1976) Biochemical genetics of the platyfishswordtail melanoma system. Prog Exp Tumor Res 20: 398

Swerdlow AJ, English J, MacKie RM, O'Doherty CJ, Hunter JAA, Clark J (1984) Benign nevi associated with high risk of melanoma. Lancet 2: 168

Taylor MR, Guerry D, Bondi EE, Shields JA, Augsburger JJ, Lusk EJ, Elder DE, Clark WH Jr., Van Horn M (1984) Intraocular melanoma is not associated with a high prevalence of cutaneous dysplastic nevi. Am J Ophthalmol 98: 478-482

Tucker MA, Misfeldt D, Coleman CN, Clark WH Jr, Rosenberg SA, Kaplan HS (1985) Cutaneous malignant melanoma following Hodgkin's disease. Ann Intern Med 102: 37-41

Vandenbark A, Greene MH, Burger D, Vetto M, Reimer RR (1979) Immune response to melanoma extracts in three melanoma prone families. JNCI 63: 1147-1151

Wallace DC, Exton LA, McLeod GRC (1971) Genetic factor in malignant melanoma. Cancer 27: 1262-1266

Wallace DC, Beardmore GL, Exton LA (1973) Familial malignant melanoma. Ann Surg 177: 15-20

*Reproducibility and Validity in the Clinical Diagnosis of the Nonfamilial Dysplastic Nevus: Work in Progress**, **

G. C. Roush, J. M. Kirkwood, M. Ernstoff, S. J. Somma, P. H. Duray, S. N. Klaus, K. S. Stenn, L. J. Titus, and A. B. Lerner

Departments of Epidemiology, Oncology, Dermatology, Pathology, and Dermatopathology, Yale University School of Medicine, Yale Melanoma Unit, New Haven, CT, USA

Introduction

An exciting development in recent years has been the documentation of a clinical syndrome characterized by familial clusters of cutaneous melanoma (CM), with members at risk for CM having multiple atypical moles (Clark et al. 1978; Greene et al. 1978; Lynch et al. 1978; Reimer et al. 1978). Persons affected by the familial dysplastic nevus syndrome (formerly known as the BK mole syndrome) have more than a 100-fold increased risk for the development of CM (Greene 1984).

While the familial dysplastic nevus syndrome is probably responsible for no more than 2%-6% of cutaneous melanomas (Anderson 1971; Duggleby et al. 1981; Kraemer et al. 1983), the nonfamilial dysplastic nevus may have wider public health implications (Kraemer et al. 1983). The prevalence of dysplastic nevus (DN) in its nonfamilial (i.e., sporadic) form is unknown. However, clinically atypical moles have been found in 2%-8% of persons from the general white population (Crutcher and Sagebiel 1984; Greene 1984; Nordlund et al. 1985; Rhodes et al. 1980). In serial examinations of patients with CM, clinically atypical nevi have been found in 30%-37% (Nordlund; Rhodes et al. 1980). From comparative data it is possible to estimate that the risk for CM in those with clinically atypical nevi is approximately 8-24 times the risk in those without atypical nevi. These data also suggest that sporadic DN might lead to at least one-third of all melanomas.

Although striking, such estimates are tentative. Prospective studies are needed to document chronology, and quantify risk for CM in those deemed to be affected by sporadic DN (Elder et al. 1982; NIH Consensus Conference 1984; Tucker et al. 1980), and assessment of the validity of clinical diagnosis is crucial to such studies. In this paper we report work in progress regarding reproducibility and validity of the clinical diagnosis of DN in the nonfamilial setting.

---

* This work is supported in part by a Preventive Oncology Award, KO7 CA 00875, from the United States National Cancer Institute

** *Abbreviations: CM,* cutaneous melanoma; *DN,* dysplastic nevus

Methods

Patients followed at the Yale Melanoma Unit were included in the study if they were newly diagnosed since January, 1983. Of 53 eligible patients, 26 were excluded initially due to ill health, infrequent clinic visits, or unwillingness to cooperate. Of the remaining 27, 26 (96%) agreed to undergo both a skin examination and biopsy of their most atypical mole. The entire skin was examined including breasts and scalp, but the anogenital surfaces were not. Examiners independently counted all nevi 3 mm or more in diameter. Also, each examiner completed a record of nevi 5 mm or more in diameter and of suggestive lesions under 5 mm in diameter, assigning coded characteristics according to the criteria for atypical nevi (Elder et al. 1982; NIH Consensus Conference 1984). These characteristics included the location of the lesion, exact size of the lesion, whether there was a macular and papular component, an irregular border, an ill-defined border, variegate color, and erythma. Up to eight lesions were so characterized for each patient. After completion of written records, the examiners confered with one another and decided on the most atypical lesion for biopsy. Photographs were taken of each lesion to be biopsied.

Two dermatopathologists read and recorded each biopsy without knowledge of the a priori clinical diagnosis. Histological criteria for diagnosis include features superimposed on junctional or compound nevus, basilar melanocytic hyperplasia with elongated rete ridges, cytologic atypia, bridging of adjacent rete ridges, lamellar and concentric dermal fibroplasia, and lymphocytes in patchy or diffuse infiltrate (NIH Consensus Conference 1984).

Results

Interobserver agreement on diagnosis of various pigmented nevi is summarized in Table 1. The diagnoses of one examiner (JMK) are compared against three other examiners re-

Table 1. Interobserver agreement in clinical diagnoses of pigmented nevi

		JMK				Agreement rates			
			JUNC,	CPD,	CONG N	All for categories		DN vs other	
		DN	NEV L	INTR		Crude	Kappa	Crude	Kappa
ME	DN	7	0	1	0	0.73	+0.58	0.91	+0.72
	JUNC, NEV L	2	6	8	0				
	CPD, INTR	1	0	19	0				
	CONG N	0	0	0	1				
SS	DN	2	0	0	0	0.63	+0.43	0.83	+0.38
	JUNC, NEV L	4	4	5	0				
	CPD, INTR	1	1	12	0				
	CONG N	0	0	0	1				
GR	DN	4	1	1	0	0.66	+0.45	0.84	+0.44
	JUNC, NEV L	3	5	8	0				
	CPD, INTR	2	0	19	0				
	CONG N	0	0	0	1				

JMK, ME, SS, and *GR* designate the four examiners. *DN,* dysplastic nevus; *JUNC,* junctional nevus; *NEV* L, nevoid lentigo; *CPD,* compound nevus; *INTR,* intradermal nevus; *CONG N,* congenital nevus

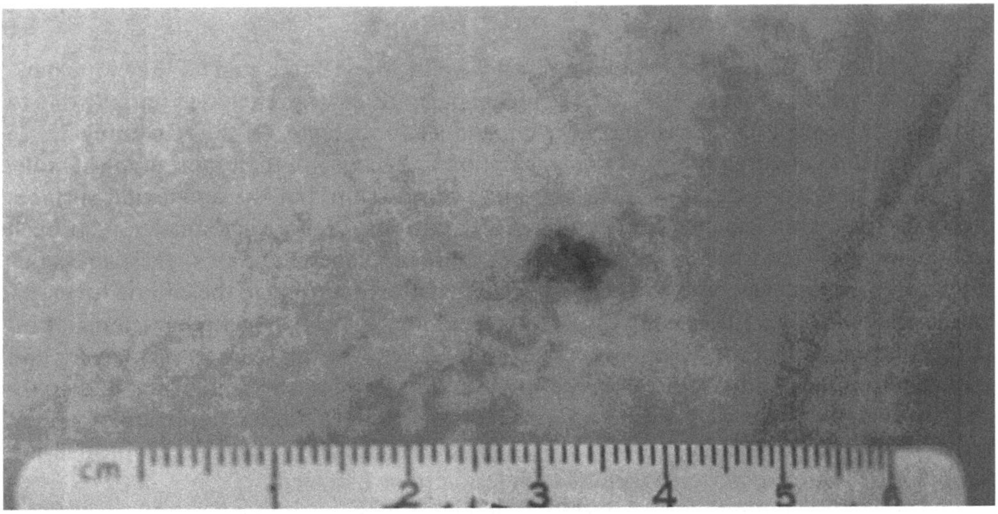

Fig. 1. A mole with longest diameter exceeding 5 mm, an irregular border, variegate color and macular component. Biopsy and histological examination confirmed the suspicion of a dysplastic nevus

Table 2. Clinical diagnosis of any one examiner versus histological diagnosis

Clinical diagnosis	Histological diagnosis		
	DN present	DN absent	
DN present	9	6	Crude agreement = 0.69 Cohen's kappa = +0.40
DN absent	2	9	Sensitivity = $^9/_{11}$ = 0.82 Specificity = $^9/_{15}$ = 0.60
	–	–	
Total	11	15	

garding four categories. The crude agreements with respect to DN range from 84% to 91%. The Kappa statistic adjusts for chance agreement, where +1.00 represents perfect agreement, zero, agreement equivalent to that expected on chance alone, and less than 1.00 disagreement.

Figure 1 demonstrates some of the clinical features of DN. The lesion is located on the trunk, and in addition to the characteristics noted in Fig. 1, parts of the border are not well defined. Prior to biopsy, each of the four examiners had recorded a clinical diagnosis of DN with moderate to high degrees of suspicion. The next question is how the a priori clinical diagnosis agrees with histopathology.

In Table 2, the a priori clinical diagnosis of one of the examiners is shown to agree with histopathology regarding the diagnosis of DN in 69% of the 26 lesions taken from each of 26 patients with CM. The sensitivity and specificity are 0.82 and 0.60, respectively.

However, these examining skills, even if verified with additional patients, must be understood in the context of their practical application in various populations wherein the true underlying prevalence of DN may vary. Table 3 indicates the positive predictive value that results from clinical skills as reflected by Table 2 and applied to three hypothetical populations. Applied to patients with CM, the predictive value is 0.58, whereas when clin-

Table 3. Positive predictive values of the clinical diagnosis of DN assuming constant sensitivity of 0.82 and specificity of 0.60 in three populations

Population	True prevalence of DN	Predictive value
General white population	0.04	0.08
Prescreened subgroup of general population	0.15	0.27
Patients with CM	0.40	0.58

ical examination skills are applied to persons from the general white population, among whom the prevalence may be 4%, the probability that the lesion given a clinical diagnosis of DN will be read as DN on histopathology is only 8%. If the same examiner evaluates an intermediate population preselected in some way (e.g., by choosing to examine persons who have risk factors for CM, such as light hair and intense adolescent sunlight exposure), the underlying prevalence of DN might be, say, 15% and the resulting predictive value approximately one-fourth.

Comment and Conclusion

Systematic biopsy of a defined target population of persons and lesions is a necessary part of achieving reproducible estimates of examining skills, because without systematic biopsy (regardless of whether or not a lesion is likely to be DN), there is no way of obtaining estimates of sensitivity and specificity. Although numbers are small, they will be augmented with enrollment of additional study subjects. We found the acceptability of biopsy among persons with melanoma to be quite high and to limit the possibility of biases owing to low rates of participation. Systematic biopsy has provided histopathological documentation of the high prevalence of DN in patients with CM (11 of 26, as shown in Table 2), a result consistent with the prevalence of clinically atypical nevi in patients with CM (Nordlund et al. 1985; Rhodes et al. 1980).

These data give some hope that careful clinical inspection of pigmented nevi can lead to the reliable diagnosis of histologically dysplastic nevi. However, the predictive value (the probability that the lesion declared to be clinically dysplastic will be dysplastic on histopathology) will be quite low in the general population unless specificity of the clinical diagnosis can be improved without sacrificing sensitivity, and unless the procedure is coupled with preselection of persons so that the underlying prevalence of DN is higher than that in the general population.

Future work will compare familial with sporadic DN with respect to clinical and histopathological features, review photographs to improve the accuracy of clinical diagnosis, grade the severity of both clinical and histological dysplasia, and quantify the risk for DN in subgroups defined by interview variables predictive of melanoma. In the present study, "clinical diagnosis of DN" refers to a suspicion which is confirmed or refuted by biopsy. This use of histopathology as the standard, although necessary in cross-sectional ascertainment of data, must ideally be replaced by a functional "gold standard," namely, the probability that a lesion designated as clinically dysplastic will be shown to progress to cutaneous melanoma, in a prospective study design (NIH Consensus Conference 1984). Such progression has already been documented in at least four lesions in which photographs of atypical nevi were obtained (Elder et al. 1982). As the diagnosis of DN becomes more secure, it will be important to describe epidemiologically the way in which sporadic DN is associated with palpable nevi on the forearms, which appear clinically normal. Palpable nevi on the arms also carry an extremely high relative risk for CM, as demonstrated elsewhere (Holman et al., this volume). If sporadic DN and palpable nevi on the arms occur in nearly the same subgroups of persons, then examination for palpable nevi might be a much simpler approach to identifying persons at high risk. A more interesting etiologic story will unfold if each of these two characteristics is shown to bear an independent relationship to risk of melanoma. The present study is obtaining data to address this question.

References

Anderson DE (1971) Clinical characteristics of the genetic variety of cutaneous melanoma in man. Cancer 28: 771-725

Clark WH Jr, Reimer RR, Greene MH, Ainsworth AM, Mastrangelo MJ (1978) Origin of familial malignant melanoma from heritable melanocytic lesions. The "BK mole syndrome". Arch Dermatol 114: 732-738

Crutcher WA, Sagebiel RW (1984) Prevalence of dysplastic naevi in a community practice (letter). Lancet 1: 729

Dubbleby WF, Stoll H, Priore RL, Greenwald P, Graham S (1981) A genetic analysis of melanoma-polygenic inheritance as a threshold trait. Am J Epidemiol 114: 63-67

Elder DE, Greene MH, Bondi EE, Clark WH Jr (1981) Acquired melanocytic nevi and melanoma: the dysplastic nevus syndrome. In: Ackerman AB (ed) Pathology of malignant melanoma. Masson, New York, 185-216

Elder DE, Kraemer KH, Greene MH, Clark WJ Jr, Guerry D (1982) The dysplastic nevus syndrome: our definition. Am J Dermatopathol 4: 455-459

Greene MH (1984) Dysplastic nevus syndrome. Hosp Pract 19: 91-108

Greene MH, Reimer RR, Clark WH Jr, Mastrangelo MJ (1978) Precursor lesions in familial melanoma. Semin Oncol 5: 85-87

Kraemer KH, Greene MG, Tarone R, Elder DE, Clark WH Jr, Guerry D (1983) Dysplastic naevi and cutaneous melanoma risk. (Letter) Lancet 2: 1076-1077

Lynch HT, Frichot B III, Lynch JF (1978) Familial atypical multiple-mole melanoma syndrome. J Med Genet 15: 352-356

NIH Consensus Conference (1984) Precursors to malignant melanoma. JAMA 251: 1864-1866

Nordlund JJ, Kirkwood J, Forget BM, Scheibner A, Albert DM, Lerner E, Milton GE (1985) Demographic study of clinically atypical (dysplastic) nevi in patients with melanoma and comparison subjects. Cancer Res 45: 1855-1861

Reimer RR, Clark WH Jr, Greene MH, Ainsworth AM, Fraumeni JF Jr. (1978) Precursor lesions in familial melanoma. A new genetic preneoplastic syndrome. JAMA 239: 744-746

Rhodes AR, Sober AJ, Mihm MC, Fitzpatrick TB (1980) Possible risk factors for primary cutaneous malignant melanoma. Clinical Res 28: 252 (abstract)

Tucker SB, Horstmann JP, Hertel B, Aranha G, Rosai J (1980) Activation of nevi in patients with malignant melanoma. Cancer 46: 822-827

Ocular Melanoma

Epidemiology of Intraocular Melanoma*

M. A. Tucker, P. Hartge, and J. A. Shields

National Cancer Insitute, Landow Building, Room 3C29, Bethesda, MD 20892, USA

Introduction

Intraocular malignant melanoma (IMM) is a relatively rare tumor, but it affects an estimated 2000 people in the United States yearly. It is the most common primary tumor of the eye in adults (Shields 1983). The incidence of IMM has been studied in descriptive studies of populations and in case reports of individuals and families. Because of the rarity of the disease, few analytic studies have been undertaken. We recently completed a case-control study of 509 IMM patients and equal number of patients with detached retinas seen by Dr. Jerry Shields at the Ocular Oncology Service of the Wills Eye Hospital in Philadelphia. We include preliminary findings from that study in this review.

Descriptive Epidemiology

Current intraocular melanoma incidence rates are 8 per million person-years in the U.S. (Cutler and Young 1975), 8 per million in Norway (Mork 1961), 7 per million in Denmark (Jensen 1963), 5 per million in Finland (Raivio 1977), and 5 per million in England (Swerdlow 1983). Intraocular melanoma incidence rates rise with increasing age and are much higher in whites than blacks; the rates for men and women appear to be fairly similar.

It seems likely that intraocular melanoma is caused by some of the same factors as cutaneous malignant melanoma, since the common cell of origin is the melanocyte and dark-skinned populations are at much lower risk of both tumors. For cutaneous melanoma, complexion and hair color are established risk factors. Eye color and hair color also appear to be related to risk of intraocular melanoma (Gallagher et al. 1985).

Approximately 10% of cutaneous melanomas are familial. Familial predisposition to intraocular melanoma has been suggested because of scattered reports of intraocular melanoma occurring in first-degree relatives of patients, and reports of cutaneous and intraocular melanoma occurring within the same individuals and families. No clear precursor lesion for intraocular melanoma has been identified, but various other medical conditions have also been associated with intraocular melanoma (nevus of Ota, neurofibromatosis, nevoid basal cell carcinoma syndrome, choroidal nevi). Several studies suggest that

* *Abbreviation: IMM,* Intraocular malignant melanoma

Recent Results in Cancer Research. Vol 102

hormone levels may affect cutaneous melanoma susceptibility, but little is known about intraocular melanoma. Ultraviolet radiation, the major environmental risk factor for cutaneous melanoma, may play a role in intraocular melanoma. Sunlight exposure was a risk factor in our recent study, but incidence rates within the U.S. and Finland are not related to latitude. Other environmental exposures have been suggested as possible causes of intraocular melanoma, including polychlorinated biphenyls, hydrazine, and dimethylsulfate.

Host Factors

Age is a strong determinant of intraocular melanoma risk, with current U.S. incidence rates rising from 0.1 per 100000 person-years at age 20 to 3.7 per 100000 person-years at age 85 (Young et al. 1981). As noted, differences in risk between men and women appear to be slight. In Finnish and American population-based studies, the incidence was slightly higher in women than men at ages below the mid-forties and slightly higher at older ages. In Danish and Norwegian population-based studies, the incidence was greater in men than in women for all ages (Jensen 1963; Mork 1961).

Race is strongly related to intraocular melanoma risk (Hakulinen et al. 1978). Scotto et al. (1976) estimated that the risk among whites was eight times greater than among blacks in the U.S. Although cutaneous melanoma is clearly associated with complexion and hair color (Elwood et al. 1984; Holman et al. 1983), this pattern has not yet been confirmed for ocular melanoma. Jensen found 69% of the normal Danish population had fair hair, while 61% of ocular melanoma patients had fair hair. There was a greater difference in color of the irides, with 61% of the normal population having fair irides (defined as blue, bluish-gray, grayish-blue, gray and greenish-gray) and 82% of the ocular melanoma patients having fair irides, with an estimated relative risk of 2.9 for people with fair irides (Jensen 1963).

Eye color, but not skin or hair color, was related to intraocular melanoma in our study. Blue-eyed subjects had the highest risk of melanoma, with an estimated relative risk of 1.7 compared with subjects with brown eyes. Unadjusted analysis showed that the patients were more likely to have fair skin, blonde or brown hair, and eastern European origin. When the analysis was adjusted for eye color, however, these differences disappeared. Conversely, adjusting for these variables did not change the risks for eye color. It is quite possible that reported eye color was a better index of actual skin color than the subject's report of skin color.

Genetic predisposition may be a factor in the development of intraocular as well as cutaneous melanoma, since there have been scattered reports of intraocular melanoma in first-degree relatives (Bowen et al. 1964; Green et al. 1978; Lynch et al. 1968; Silcock 1892; Tasman 1970). In our study, however, only 4 of 3422 (0.1%) first-degree relatives of patients had eye cancers, suggesting that familial occurrence probably accounts for very little of the disease. Unlike cutaneous melanomas, which are frequently multiple, bilateral intraocular melanomas are quite rare. It has been estimated that one case of bilateral choroidal melanoma occurs every 18 years in the U.S. (Shammas and Watze 1977).

Intraocular melanoma has been reported as a double primary with cutaneous melanoma (Paton and Thomas 1959), with ovarian cancer (Mullaney et al. 1984), and with breast cancer (Harvey and Brinton 1985). In our study, although the numbers are small and did not reach statistical significance, there is a two-fold risk of intraocular melanoma after ovarian tumors. There was no increased risk after breast cancer.

Nevus of Ota (oculodermal melanocytosis) is a recognized risk factor for both intraocular melanoma (Font et al. 1967; Halasa 1970) and cutaneous melanoma, but this risk has been difficult to quantitate. Intraocular melanoma has also been reported as part of the constellations of tumors which occur in neurofibromatosis (Gartner 1940), an autosomal dominant phakomatosis, and in nevoid basal cell carcinoma syndrome (Kedem et al. 1970), an autosomal dominant mesodermal abnormality.

Iris nevi may be related to development of intraocular melanoma, but in one study equal numbers of iris nevi were found in the eye that developed intraocular melanoma and the unaffected eye (Michelson and Shields 1977). Posterior choroidal nevi have also been thought to be precursor lesions, but Ganley and Comstock estimated that if intraocular melanoma arose only from choroidal nevi, the average annual incidence of intraocular melanoma would be 21 per 100000 persons with choroidal nevi (Ganley and Comstock 1973). In our study, subjects with iris melanoma were approximately three times as likely as controls to have iris nevi, but not choroidal nevi. The nevi which were recorded in the medical records were separate from the tumor itself. Conversely, we found no significant association between choroidal nevi and choroidal melanoma. This may be because iris nevi are multiple more often than are choroidal nevi, and if a person has a single precursor lesion, it may in fact be the nevus that becomes a melanoma. Alternatively, there may be no association between choroidal nevi and choroidal melanoma.

Recently, a precursor lesion for cutaneous melanoma, the dysplastic nevus, has been characterized (Clark et al. 1978, 1984; Greene et al. 1985). These lesions identify individuals who are at high risk for both familial and sporadic melanoma. Two kindreds with cutaneous melanoma, intraocular melanoma, and dysplastic nevus syndrome have been described, but in these families the associations of cutaneous melanoma, dysplastic nevi, and intraocular melanoma appeared to be coincidental (Greene et al. 1983). A subsequent evaluation of a small series of intraocular melanoma patients revealed that intraocular melanoma patients had a 4.5% prevalence of dysplastic nevi, as against a 41% prevalence of dysplastic nevi in patients with sporadic cutaneous melanoma (Taylor et al. 1984). In our study, subjects were asked specifically about certain skin conditions possibly associated with intraocular melanoma, including skin melanoma, moles, other skin cancers, birthmarks such as the nevus of Ota, congenital nevi, café-au-lait spots, or other skin conditions such as psoriasis.

Patients with intraocular melanoma were twice as likely as controls to report prominent moles. At this point, we do not know whether these are true nevi, actinic keratoses, or other pigmented lesions. The numbers were very small, and the risks did not reach statistical significance, but cutaneous melanoma was slightly more common (relative risk = 1.6) in the intraocular melanoma cases. There was no difference in birthmarks or pigmentary abnormalities. In our study, cases were four times as likely as controls to have psoriasis. This statistically significant excess was not due to treatment with psoralens and ultraviolet radiation and persisted even in those who did not have this therapy.

The observation that we found no association with birthmarks or pigmentary abnormalities may be explained by the difference in data between case reports or clinical series, and questionnaire data. The data from clinical observation are much more accurate and precise than data obtained from a questionnaire. Even if there is a very high risk associated with the nevus of Ota, ocular melanocytosis, neurofibromatosis, or any other condition, it may not be found in a case-control study, simply because of reporting. Similarly, as noted above, "moles" according to the general population may be actinic keratoses, pigmented basal cell carcinomas, true nevi, hemangiomas, etc.

Environmental Factors

Ultraviolet radiation from sun exposure, the major environmental risk factor for cutaneous melanoma, has not been thought to be strongly related to intraocular melanoma risk, since it does not show the strong association with latitude characteristics of cutaneous melanoma (Lee 1982). For example, no latitude differences for intraocular melanoma have been found in the United States (Scotto et al. 1976) or Finland (Raivio 1977), or in a comparison of multiple countries (Hakulinen et al. 1978). It should be noted, however, that an examination of the effect of latitude in the United States is somewhat confused by the association of ethnicity and hence coloring with latitude (Morin et al. 1984). In the United States, tumor registries in the north include more fair-skinned, blue-eyed populations than the southern registries do. In addition, although the incidence of cutaneous melanoma is increasing rapidly, which has been attributed to increasing sun exposure (Lee 1982), the incidence rates of intraocular melanoma have remained stable over time (Scotto et al. 1976; Strickland and Lee 1981; Swerdlow 1983).

Previous U.S. studies have shown a difference in laterality by sex with an increase in left eye melanoma in men and right eye melanoma in women (Keller 1973; Scotto et al. 1976). It was hypothesized that this might relate to driving habits in the U.S., with the left eye being exposed to more sun and/or pollutants in males, and the right in females (Scotto et al. 1976). In our study, there was no difference in laterality in either sex.

Our study findings suggest that sunlight exposure does increase IMM risk, judging by differences between cases and controls in birthplace, freckling, sunbathing, sunlamp use, and eye protection (Tucker et al. 1985). Patients were three times more likely to be born in the southern states than controls, after adjustment for eye color, age, and sex. To exclude the possibility that referral bias accounted for the excess of cases born in the south, we looked at those study subjects living in greater Philadelphia at the time of diagnosis and found the same increased risk. Living in the south for a long time was less important than being born in the south as a predictor of melanoma risk. This is consistent with the observation that the lens filters most ultraviolet radiation by the adult years (Zigman 1983). Only a small number of study subjects had lived in the tropics and subtropics for 5 years or more, but they, too, showed a striking elevation in risk (RR = 4) (Tucker et al. 1985).

Freckles are an index of both sensitivity and exposure to sun. The cases were slightly more likely to have over 25 freckles (RR = 1.4). They were also more likely to use sunlamps (RR = 1.4), with some evidence of increasing risk with increasing frequency of use ($P = 0.10$). This relationship was not confounded by the effect of psoriasis. Study subjects with intraocular melanoma were more likely to sunbathe (RR = 1.4), but frequency of sunbathing did not appear to be related to risk (Tucker et al. 1985).

Eye protection was also associated with lowered intraocular melanoma risk in our study. Compared with subjects who almost always used eye protection when in the sun, those who did not had a 60% increase in risk (95% CI = 1.0–2.2), but there was no gradation in risk depending on whether the subjects wore protection occasionally, rarely, or never. Another form of eye shading that might protect against intraocular melanoma is corrective lens use. More patients with detached retina wore glasses most of the time than did patients with intraocular melanoma (64% vs 52%) (Tucker et al. 1985). Because of the poorer visual acuity of the patients with detached retina, we used a second control group with visual acuity similar to the cases and found a 20% reduction in risk, which was not statistically significant.

Not all indicators of sunlight exposure were related to intraocular melanoma risk in our study. For example, there was no difference in the total amount of leisure time that patients and controls spent outdoors, but there were differences in the types of outdoor leisure. Gardening as a hobby was associated with an increased risk of ocular melanoma (RR = 1.6), which was not attributable to fertilizer, pesticide, or herbicide use. Cases were also more likely to spend increased amounts of time out in the sun during vacations compared to everyday living (RR = 1.3). Adjusting for the length of vacation did not change the estimated risks (Tucker et al. 1985).

Social class was examined in a Finnish study as a rough occupational index, but the distribution of intraocular melanoma by social class was identical to the general population (Raivio 1977). In Denmark, there was a similar distribution of occupations in the case group and the general population, except for an increased percentage in domestic work and, possibly, construction work. The increased percentage of domestic workers was attributed to differences in employment reporting among housewives between the study questionnaire and population census questionnaire (Jensen 1963). In our study, the distribution of occupations was very similar among cases and controls. Time spent working outdoors also was similar among cases and controls. We examined the occupations with high ultraviolet exposure, such as welding, construction work, or farming, in which risk of intraocular melanoma might be elevated. Welders and construction workers had elevated risks according to these data, but farmers did not. Subjects who said they worked under bare fluorescent lights were at slightly increased risk. None of these estimates of occupation-specific relative risk was stable, because of the small numbers of workers in each category.

Exogenous estrogen may be a factor for cutaneous melanoma (Beral et al. 1977; Danforth et al. 1982; Helmrich et al. 1983; Holly et al. 1983), but the issue is controversial. In this study, there was no difference in duration of use or type of oral contraceptives between cases and controls. Ever having been pregnant was associated with an increaed risk of melanoma (RR = 1.4), but there was no increasing risk with increasing parity. There was also no effect of age at first pregnancy or latency between last pregnancy and diagnosis. The age at menarche and age at menopause were similar in the two groups. Postmenopausal estrogen use was associated with a significantly increased risk of melanoma, with dose response reaching a threefold risk in those who took postmenopausal estrogens for 6 years or longer.

Chemical exposures have been implicated in the etiology of both cutaneous and intraocular melanoma. Cutaneous melanoma has beem associated with exposure to polychlorinated biphenyls and other industrial toxins (Bahn et al. 1976). Intraocular melanoma has occurred in excess in chemical plant workers in West Virginia, possibly due to hydrazine and dimethylsulfate exposure (Albert et al. 1980). Our preliminary analysis suggests an increased risk associated with working in the plastics industry or with the manufacture of plastics. Patients were more likely to be exposed to chemicals and radiation, as well as pesticides, fertilizers, and paints. There were no significant effects of either alcohol or tobacco use.

Future studies need to confirm and further refine these results, particularly to clarify the mode and intensity of ultraviolet exposure, and the effects of early life and intermittent ultraviolet exposure on the risks of IMM. In this way, it should be possible to lower the incidence of ocular melanoma, which is presently a serious cause of morbidity and vision loss.

References

Albert DM, Puliafito CA, Fulton AB, et al. (1980) Increased incidence of choroidal melanoma occurring in a single population of chemical workers. Am J Ophthalmol 89: 323-337
Bahn AK, Rosenwaike I, Herrman H, et al. (1976) Melanoma after exposure to PCBs. N Engl J Med 295: 450
Beral V, Rancharan S, Faris R (1977) Malignant melanoma and oral contraceptive use among women in California. Br J Cancer 36: 804-809
Bowen SF, Brady H, Jones VL (1964) Malignant melanoma of eye occurring in two successive generations. Arch Ophthalmol 71: 805-806
Clark WH Jr, Reimer RR, Greene MH, et al. (1978) Origin of familial melanoma from heritable melanocytic lesions: the B-K mole syndrome. Arch Dermatol 114: 732-738
Clark WH Jr, Elder DE, Guerry D, et al. (1984) A study of tumor progression: the precursor lesions of superficial spreading and nodular melanoma. Hum Pathol 15: 1147-1165
Cutler SJ, Young JL Jr (eds) (1975) Third national cancer survey: incidence data. Natl Cancer Inst Monogr 41
Danforth DN, Russell N, MCBride CM (1982) Hormonal status of patients with primary malignant melanoma: a review of 313 cases. South Med J 75: 661-664
Elwood JM, Gallagher RP, Hill GB, et al. (1984) Pigmentation and skin reaction to sun as risk factors for cutaneous melanoma: Western Canada melanoma study. Br Med J 288: 99-102
Font RL, Reynolds AM, Zimmerman LF (1967) Diffuse malignant melanoma of the iris in the nevus of Ota. Arch Ophthalmol 77: 513-518
Gallagher RP, Elwood JM, Rootman J, et al. (1985) Risk factors for ocular melanoma: Western Canada melanoma study. JNCI 74: 775-778
Ganley JP, Comstock GW (1973) Benign nevi and malignant melanomas of the choroid. Am J Ophthalmol 76: 19-25
Gartner S (1940) Malignant melanoma of the choroid and von Recklinghausen's disease. Am J Ophthalmol 23: 73-78
Green EJ, Hong WK, Everett JR, et al. (1978) Familial intraocular malignant melanoma: a case report. Cancer 41: 2481-2483
Greene MH, Sanders RJ, Chu FC, et al. (1983) The familial occurrence of cutaneous melanoma intraocular melanoma, and the dysplastic nevus syndrome. Am J Ophthalmol 96: 238-245
Greene MH, Clark WH Jr, Tucker MA, et al. (1985) Acquired precursors of cutaneous malignant melanoma - the familial dysplastic nevus syndrome. N Engl J Med 312: 91-98
Hakulinen T, Tempo L, Saxon E (1978) Cancer of the eye: a review of trends and differentials. World Health Stat Q 31: 143-158
Halasa A (1970) Malignant melanoma in a bilaterial nevus of Ota. Arch Ophthalmol 84: 176-179
Harvey EB, Brinton LA (1985) Second cancer following cancer of the breast in Connecticut, 1935-1982. In: Boice JD Jr, Fraumeni JF Jr, Curtis RE, et al (eds) Multiple primary cancer in Connecticut and Denmark. Natl Cancer Inst Monogr 68: 99-112
Helmrich S, Rosenberg L, Shapiro S, et al. (1983) Malignant melanoma and oral contraceptive use. Am J Epidemiol 118: 417 (abstract)
Holly EA, Weiss NS, Liff JM (1983) Cutaneous melanoma in relation to exogeneous hormones and reproductive factors. JNCI 70: 827-831
Holman CDJ, Armstrong BK, Heenan PJ (1983) A theory of the etiology and pathogenesis of human cutaneous melanoma. JNCI 71: 651-656
Jenson O (1963) Malignant melanomas of the uvea in Denmark 1943-1952: a clinical, histopathological and prognostic study. Acta Ophthalmol [Suppl] 75: 1-220
Kedem A, Even-Paz Z, Freund M (1970) Basal cell nevus syndrome associated with malignant melanoma of the iris. Dermatologica 140: 99-106
Keller AZ (1973) Histology, survivorship and related factors in the epidemiology of eye cancers. Am J Epidemiol 97: 386-393
Lee JAH (1982) Melanoma In: Schottenfeld D, Fraumeni JF Jr (eds) Cancer epidemiology and prevention. Saunders, Philadelphia, pp 984-993

Lynch HT, Anderson DE, Krush AJ (1968) Heredity and intraocular malignant melanoma. Cancer 21: 119-129
Michelson JB, Shields JA (1977) Relationship of iris nevi to malignant melanoma of the uvea. Am J Ophthalmol 83: 694-696
Morin M, Pickle L, Mason TJ (1984) Geographic patterns of ethnic groups in the United States. Am J Public Health 74: 133-139
Mork T (1961) Malignant neoplasms of the eye in Norway: incidence, treatment, and prognosis. Acta Ophthalmol 39: 824-831
Mullaney J, Mooney D, O'Connor M, McDonald GSA (1984) Bilateral ovarian carcinoma with bilateral uveal melanoma. Br J Ophthalmol 68: 261-267
Paton D, Thomas LB (1959) Simultaneous occurrence of primary malignant melanomas of the eye and the skin. Arch Ophthalmol 62: 645-652
Pfingst AO, Graves S (1921) Melanosarcoma of the choroid occurring in brothers. Arch Ophthalmol 50: 431-439
Raivio I (1977) Uveal melanoma in Finland: an epidemiological, clinical, histological and prognostic study. Acta Ophthalmol [suppl] 133: 1-64
Scotto J, Fraumeni JF, Lee JAH (1976) Melanomas of the eye and other noncutaneous sites: epidemiologic aspects. JNCI 56: 489-491
Shammas HF, Watze RC (1977) Bilateral choroidal melanomas: case report and incidence. Arch Ophthalmol 95: 617-623
Shields JA (1983) Introduction to melanocytic tumors of the uvea. In: Shields JA (ed) Diagnosis and management of intraocular tumors. Mosby, St. Louis, pp 65-82
Silcock AO (1892) Hereditary sarcoma of the eyeball in three generations. Br Med J 1: 1079
Strickland D, Lee JAH (1981) Melanomas of eye: stability of rates. Am J Epidemiol 113: 700-702
Swerdlow AJ (1983) Epidemiology of melanoma of the eye in the Oxford region, 1952-78. Br J Cancer 47: 311-313
Tasman W (1970) Familial intraocular melanoma. Trans Am Acad Ophthalmol Otolaryngol 74: 955-958
Taylor ME, Guerry D, Bondi EE, et al (1984) Lack of association between intraocular melanoma and cutaneous dysplastic nevi. Am J Ophthalmol 98: 478-482
Tucker MA, Shields JA, Hartge P, et al (1985) Sunlight exposure as risk factor for intraocular malignant melanoma. N Engl J Med 313: 789-792
Young JL, Percy CL, Asire AJ (eds) (1981) Surveillance, epidemiology an end results: incidence and mortality data 1973-1977. Natl Cancer Inst Monogr 57
Zigman S (1983) The role of sunlight in human cataract formation. Surv Ophthalmol 27: 317-325

Subject Index

MIX
Papier aus verantwortungsvollen Quellen
Paper from responsible sources
FSC® C105338

If you have any concerns about our products,
you can contact us on
ProductSafety@springernature.com

In case Publisher is established outside the EU,
the EU authorized representative is:
Springer Nature Customer Service Center GmbH
Europaplatz 3, 69115 Heidelberg, Germany

Printed by Libri Plureos GmbH
in Hamburg, Germany